S0-BDL-882

Staying Slim the Natural Way

The **BOOKS 2000** series has been developed to help Americans understand the exciting discoveries and developments and solve the day-to-day problems that will confront us all in the challenging years between now and the year 2000.

Other titles in this series include:

Buyer Beware: How To Be a Smart Shopper

How To Save on Taxes: A Year-Round Plan

Pot, Pills, & Powders: The Truth About Drugs

Household Hints

I Am an American

Stretch Your House: Easy Space-Saving Ideas

Easy Home Repairs

What Are the Odds?

Living With Your Heart

BOOKS 2000...THE BOOKS THAT LOOK AHEAD

Staying Slim
the Natural Way

Virginia Livingston

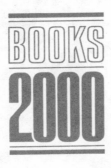

NEW YORK • 1972

Copyright © 1972 by Western Publishing Company, Inc.,
850 Third Avenue, New York, New York 10022.
All rights reserved.

BOOKS 2000 is a trademark of Western Publishing Company, Inc.

Library of Congress Catalog Card Number: 71–162417

Printed in the United States of America.

Foreword

America is the most overfed, overweight nation in the world. Yet a shocking number of Americans—including the rich!—are appallingly undernourished.

Today, more than ever, we need to preserve every scrap of energy and vitality we can to survive the pressures of space-age living—not to mention the toll polluted air and water takes on our bodies.

Our families, friends, lovers, and employers demand that we look young and stay slim. Moreover, we *must* stay slim if we are to have any chance of avoiding heart disease.

To do this we must reduce our calory intake *but* maintain and often increase our intake of vitamins and minerals.

Is it possible? Yes, and in *Staying Slim the Natural Way,* Virginia Livingston—who has been in the thick of the nutrition controversy since early childhood—shows you how easy and satisfying it is to recapture your youthful appearance without jeopardizing your health.

Michael Dorn *for* BOOKS 2000

Contents

1 What Is the Natural Way?

LET'S GET THIN and stay thin.

But let's do it without going on a painful, rigid exercise plan that neither you nor I have any serious intention of following for any length of time.

Let's do it without buying a houseful of expensive "diet" and "low calory" foods that have warnings on their labels that read like the danger warnings on a cigarette package.

Let's get thin and stay thin without going onto a lot of faddish, crackpot diets that do as much harm as good—diets that claim to take 10 pounds off in one week (*but that you're warned not to stay on for longer than one week because of the harm done to your body*).

Let's get thin and stay thin the natural way.

What is the natural way?

First let's take a look at *what is not the natural way*. There is nothing natural about forcing yourself to eat the great variety of unusual food products that have become so well-known thanks to the current popularity of health-food stores and restaurants and the macrobiotic fad. Health-fad foods are not necessarily natural foods. Foods such as yogurt, wheat germ, brewer's yeast, soy beans, raw liver—all these are certainly good for you. They are high in proteins and vitamins and often low in calories and fat.

But if you don't like them, if you can't learn to like them, *you simply are not going to eat them,* and you'll be right back where you started from, gaining weight and feeling more guilty than ever.

There is nothing natural about eating foods you don't like—regardless of how naturally those foods are grown or how healthful they are.

There is no reason for you to patronize a health-food store if you don't want to. Your local supermarket is well stocked with a great variety of fresh fruits, vegetables, and meats that you already know and like, that are low in fats and calories, and that can give you all the vitamins you need and want.

The trick is to know what the good foods are, which are low in calories, and how to prepare them properly. The trick is to avoid high-calory foods and the uninteresting ways of preparing low-calory ones.

There is nothing natural about doing exercises that are painful, exhausting, difficult, and serve little purpose other than to train you for the Olympics.

Why torture yourself? There are many simple, painless, *natural* exercises that you can do to keep your muscles firm and your body in good condition. These exercises are so easy, they come so *naturally,* that you will soon be only barely aware that you are doing them.

Forget past failures

You have just turned a new page to take weight off and keep it off. Very possibly you have lost hundreds of pounds in the past 10 years—and gained back in just a few weeks more than you ever lost.

Forget past failures. Learn the secret of selection for staying thin. Nature is an abundant supplier of nourishing, delicious, low-calorie food.

The natural road to success

If you need to shed ten pounds or fifty, you must have a comfortably realistic method that enables you to lose weight without altering your life style. Achieving this goal requires only that you change the emphasis on the *types of foods you eat and exercises you take*.

Nature's secrets

It's natural to be thin. The best way to stay thin is the natural way. Nature has all kinds of secrets for getting those extra pounds off and keeping them off. You owe it to yourself to find out what they are. You'll live longer, be happier, look younger and more attractive.

Here, briefly, is Nature's basic secret for weight control:

- Eat only the low-calorie foods that you like; do only those exercises that you enjoy doing.
- But select those foods and exercises from Nature's private list of fat fighters and youth preservers.

This book has been designed to give you a thorough understanding of nature's built-in remedy for overweight . . . to acquaint you thoroughly with that list so that you will soon know immediately which foods are your friends and which foods are deadly enemies.

For starters, let's take a close look at that food-hungry maniac, the Carboholic . . . and *his* drug: high-fat, sugar, and starch food.

2 Kick the Carboholic Habit

WHAT IS A CARBOHOLIC? Are you one? If you're overweight, you may be. If you've been dieting for years, taking off three pounds one week only to gain back five the next, you probably *are*.

Do you try every fad diet that comes along, hoping that at last you've found the answer? Have you tried dozens of diets that worked. . . really worked . . . and then gone off them simply because you didn't like what you were eating and couldn't resist the temptation to return to your former food choices?

Then you probably are a carboholic. You have an ir-resistible desire to overstuff yourself with foods. The desire may stem from emotional causes, from social causes, from sheer boredom. In the end it doesn't matter. *You're eating compulsively and you've got to stop*.

How serious is carboholism?

Let me give you an extreme example. I have a friend who is a chronic carboholic. He was born with a silver spoon in his mouth—a rich family, a long line of illustrous ances-tors. He was given the best education. He was handsome and charming. A great career lay before him.

But somewhere along the line something went wrong. I don't know what—perhaps just space-age pressures.

10

He took to eating compulsively, as the alcoholic turns to liquor. That silver spoon turned into a shovel.

In a few short years he was transformed from the fair-haired young man of the State Department into a fat, unattractive failure. His career was ruined and before long he turned to alcohol, too. He stuffed himself with food to forget his failures, and drank to forget his weight.

His money didn't help him. If anything it hurt. He didn't really have to work. When he was so fat and so drunk that he was at death's door, his doctors simply sent him away to a fancy funny farm for a few months, where he went on the wagon, lost 10 or 20 or 50 pounds, and took the baths.

When he left the farm and returned to his empty life it was only a matter of weeks before he abandoned his diet. The pounds started creeping back. He couldn't help himself. And then he started drinking. The vicious circle.

He is still on this same routine today. He may never get off it until it kills him.

Why? Because he's never faced the fact that he is a carboholic. All the doctors and money in the world can't help him. Like the alcoholic, the carboholic can only help himself. Drugs and spas provide only temporary relief. And may do more harm than good.

That is an extreme example. Let's look at the "average" carboholic.

Mildred Jackson recently turned 30. Until a few years ago she never had to worry about her weight. Even after producing two children she could eat as much as she pleased. She didn't even think about weighing herself.

Two years ago she was shocked when she found she couldn't get into her swimming suit. Of course she was vaguely aware that she had put on a pound or two. Her

11

husband had been kidding her about it all winter—always adding that he liked her better this way. Hadn't she always been a little too thin?

Nevertheless, Mildred decided to take a few pounds off. She would have cottage cheese for lunch. Skip the second martini. She wasn't overweight. Certainly not. But it would be nice to get back into that bikini.

It didn't work. Instead of losing she continued to gain. At 30 she was 12 pounds overweight. Her doctor advised her to shed a few pounds but she couldn't. Finally she decided that she *shouldn't*. After all, she really wasn't eating any more than she ever had. It must be glandular. It is natural for the body to gain weight as it gets older, she told herself. Crash diets didn't work for her. Why fight nature? She resigned herself to being fat. *She had become a carboholic*.

Mildred's theory was all wet—even though she no longer went swimming.

It is not natural for the body to gain weight as it gets older. The truth of the matter is that by the time the body reaches the age of 25 it requires about one percent less food each year to maintain the basic functions such as breathing, digesting, heart action, and generally getting through the day.

Unless you reduce the amount of food you take in at this time of life—or increase your physical activity—you are bound to gain weight. The diet that keeps you svelte at twenty can make you chubby at thirty and downright fat at forty.

What are the dangers of carboholism?

Mildred is in trouble. When you're even 10 pounds overweight you run the risk of dying five or 10 years sooner.

If you're 20 pounds overweight, your mortality rate is 10 percent above average.

If you're 30 pounds overweight, your mortality rate is 25 percent above average.

If you're 50 pounds overweight, your mortality rate is 50–75 percent above average!

You run the risk of diabetes, digestive disorders, high blood pressure, and heart disease.

The calory: What is it?

Don't be a carboholic. The first thing to do to avoid this disease is to learn a few basic facts about your friend—or enemy—the calory.

To tell you what calories are doesn't mean that you have to count them. Calories *do* count—but counting them won't do you a bit of good unless you know what to do with your arithmetic.

The calory is a unit of measurement of energy that comes from everything we eat and much of what we drink. The food and beverages—and therefore calories—that we eat and drink are made up of:

- Protein.
- Fat.
- Carbohydrate.

Each of us uses a certain number of calories a day to sustain life. If you eat more calories than your body needs, you gain weight and store fat in your body. If you eat fewer calories than your body needs, your body will convert the existing fat to fuel and you will lose weight.

The importance of protein

You've been hearing about the value of protein and high protein diets since you first worried about your weight.

Is it really true that protein is the dieter's best friend? If so, why?

You bet it's true. Protein not only keeps you from getting fat—it actually goes to work to burn up the fat you've already got.

An ounce of fat contains 225 calories. An ounce of protein contains 113 calories.

When you eat an ounce of fat it turns into more fat in your body. When you eat an ounce of protein it starts producing energy in your body—so much that *you burn up 130 to 140 calories for every 113 that you eat!*

This is one of nature's most marvelous secrets.

Jonathan Winters, the hilarious television comic, has had a long struggle with weight. One of his jokes is about celery. He used to say "Celery has minus two calories. Minus, because it doesn't have any to start with and you burn up two chewing it."

The truth is, a stalk of celery has *minus 7½ calories!* It has five calories to start out with (plus vitamin C, niacin, iron, and other needed minerals). The protein in it causes it to burn 12½ calories in your body. So: *minus 7½*—and that's not counting the calories you burn up chewing it!

How many calories do you need?

Fewer than you think . . . if you've been using old-fashioned weight charts to determine your ideal weight.

Until very recently, ideal weight charts were based on the *average weight* of the *average American—who was usually overweight!* Because he was "average," he was considered to be "ideal."

New weight chart for the seventies

Today doctors agree that the "average" is much too heavy.

Look over the revised chart below and see where you stand. The weights listed are within 10 percent of being ideal for healthy adults. The margin is allowed for the differences in heavy, light, or medium bone structure.

If you weigh more than these ideal weights you may still not be a real fatty.

A look in the mirror or a side glance in the passing store window is the way to tell. Does your jacket have that strained, pleated look? Is your dress pulled tight around your stomach and hips? Unless you visit your tailor or dressmaker often, you have this look when you've gained a few pounds.

What You Should Weigh Undressed
and Unfed in the A.M.

WOMEN

Height (with 2″ heels)	Small Frame	Medium Frame	Large Frame
4ft 10in	92–98	96–107	104–119
4ft 11in	94–101	98–110	106–122
5ft 0in	96–104	101–113	109–125
5ft 1in	99–107	104–116	112–128
5ft 2in	102–110	107–119	115–131
5ft 3in	105–113	110–122	118–134
5ft 4in	108–116	113–126	121–138
5ft 5in	111–119	116–130	125–142
5ft 6in	114–123	120–135	129–146
5ft 7in	118–127	124–139	133–150
5ft 8in	122–131	128–143	137–154
5ft 9in	126–135	132–147	141–158
5ft 10	130–140	136–151	145–163
5ft 11in	134–144	140–155	149–168
6ft 0in	138–148	144–159	153–173

continued on next page

MEN

Height (1″ heels)	Small Frame	Medium Frame	Large Frame
5ft 2in	112–120	118–129	126–141
5ft 3in	115–123	121–133	129–144
5ft 4in	118–126	124–136	132–148
5ft 5in	121–129	127–139	135–152
5ft 6in	124–133	130–143	138–156
5ft 7in	128–137	134–147	142–161
5ft 8in	132–141	138–152	147–166
5ft 9in	136–145	142–156	151–170
5ft 10in	140–150	146–160	155–174
5ft 11in	144–154	150–165	159–179
6ft 0in	148–158	154–170	164–184
6ft 1in	152–162	158–175	168–189
6ft 2in	156–167	162–180	173–194
6ft 3in	160–171	167–185	178–199
6ft 4in	164–175	172–190	182–204

Prepared by the Metropolitan Life Insurance Co. from data of the Build and Blood Pressure Study, *1959, Society of Actuaries.*

Unless you are an active athlete, you won't accept an exercise program that is like training for the Olympics. There is little enough time in the day for just the usual activities.

But you can sneak in all sorts of easy, painless exercises—and hardly be aware that you're doing them—simply by becoming a little more aware of the way your muscles feel and function as you pass your normal day. These exercises are not designed specifically to help you shed pounds. They are designed to keep your muscles and skin firm and wrinkle-free as you shed pounds the natural way—by eating only the delicious, nutritious foods that nature has created to fight fat.

Don't be a carboholic. Live longer, be happier. Go on the wagon today—the food wagon. It's the natural way.

3   Think Thin...Be Thin

IT'S NATURAL to be thin. Animals are thin. (I mean non-domesticated animals living in their natural environment. That fat tabby cat you know, that obese cocker spaniel—they are not living in a natural state. They are subject to many of the pressures you are, and are not healthy pets.)

One of the first things to do when you've decided to kick carboholism once and for all is to learn to think thin. It is one of the greatest aids in weight reduction.

Thinking thin is *not-thinking about fat*—about *your* fat, or about fatty foods, rich foods that quickly add ugly pounds.

Thinking thin does not mean pretending that calories don't exist, or being deceived by lies about them—as so many people were when told by a popular book that calories don't count. (That book was discredited legally and medically because it was untrue, and the people who followed its instructions were gaining weight.)

Calories *do* count. But when you think thin, *you* forget about counting them. It's unnecessary and a bore. And you're a bore when you keep talking about how many calories you're eating or not eating today.

When you look up the number of calories in a certain food (such as chocolate cake or cream pie) you're only hurting yourself. Your mind is then turned in the direction

17

of these high-calory foods and you picture them so vividly that you may even start salivating, and you can't resist them.

You start thinking about fatty foods and soon, fat conscious, you begin to picture yourself as fat and unattractive, and thus start the "feeling-hopelessly-fat" cycle going. That is *thinking fat*.

Don't. I have a friend in Chicago, an interior decorator, who was hooked on thinking fat. When she wanted to buy a new frock she would go to a chic boutique and head directly for the full-length, three-way mirrors. Then she would wallow in misery. *No,* she would say, *I'm too fat. First I've got to find a good crash diet.*

Then she would start musing about all the goodies that she would have to give up. She would feel worse and worse until she rushed out of the boutique and into the nearest Howard Johnson's for a hot fudge sundae.

If she hadn't started thinking about FAT, she wouldn't have started associating the fat with the foods that were responsible for it. She continued thinking about them until she couldn't wait to get more to make her feel less sad about their effects. She ate sweets to forget her fat like an alcoholic drinks whisky to forget his hangover.

Pleasure—and wayward parents

To think thin you must become aware of the many things . . . in addition to fuel for your body's engine . . . that food means to you.

One of the things it means is pleasure. There is nothing wrong with pleasure, and food is a source of enormous pleasure to all of us. How to enjoy it without becoming fat is discussed at length in Chapter 4—"The Sensuous Dieter."

Food also serves as a reward and a consolation. Too often,

high-calory foods such as cookies, cake, and candy were given to us by our parents throughout childhood to console us for a disappointment, or to reward us for an achievement.

If you realize that certain foods have continued to have this meaning to you, you can learn to substitute other kinds of treats that have nothing to do with food.

You're not a kid anymore. It's time to reward yourself with an adult reward and console yourself like an adult.

Think about some little thing that you would very much like to have or to do—an unusual vacation or weekend, something extravagant for the house, a fascinating novel, "the works" at your local beauty salon or barber.

Then figure out a way of getting or doing it. File the suggestions away and the next time that you are disappointed or hurt, or have done a very good job, go to the file and give yourself the new reward or consolation. *Reach for an idea instead of a sweet!*

Know yourself, like yourself

I can't say it too often: To think thin, stop thinking of yourself as fat. Stop accepting yourself as fat. But don't stop accepting yourself altogether.

It is essential that you like yourself. Like yourself enough to think of yourself as being slim and attractive. Don't stand looking at those bulges in the mirror; don't squeeze those bags of fat around your belly until you're ready to weep. Don't start the depression cycle.

Picture yourself as looking as slim and attractive in your clothes as the most attractive person you know.

Exciting thin foods for the seventies

One of the roadblocks to thinking thin in the past was the feeling that everything good to eat is fattening. It isn't true.

In the last 10 years an enormous amount of time, money, and scientific investigation has been devoted to the selection and combination of low-calory menus and recipes. Anyone willing to try them will find them delicious.

Read the chapters on low-calory foods, and the natural ways to exercise. Familiarize yourself with the exercises by reading them over a number of times before you go to sleep. Be able to call to mind many of the low-calory foods easily. While you are lying in bed, picture yourself doing the exercises as you walk, sit, or stand through the day. Do the facial exercises as you lie in bed.

Think of which muscles you use: Tense them and stretch them just a little (not enough to greatly increase circulation). It is a pleasant sensation. All movement is exercise. Your old horror of exercise will vanish.

Think of the elegant thin foods, the "in" foods. Whip up some of my low-calory butter, sour cream, mayonnaise, or hollandaise. Try some of the recipes for creamy, low-calory soups.

At first try just the recipes that appeal to you. Then try them all. You will find that they are just as delicious as your former choices. Soon you will wonder how you were ever able to eat those greasy, rich, unnatural foods.

You will begin to change your attitude toward what you think you like. You will have hurdled the psychological barrier and will be on the positive road of *thinking thin*.

4 The Sensuous Dieter

EVERYONE WHO LIKES FOOD is a sensuous dieter. We like the pleasure that food gives to each of our five senses. And why not? Using our senses for pleasure is one of the great ways of enjoying life. It has taken man several thousand years to develop the many ways to achieve maximum sensual satisfaction.

Then what's wrong?

Brillat-Savarin, the great French gourmet, said in his *Physiologie du Gout:* "In compelling man to eat that he may live, nature gives him an appetite to invite him and pleasure to reward him."

To taste is a great gift of nature. *If you are overweight, it is not because your tastebuds are keener than most people's* (although if you are a nonsmoker and a light drinker, you may have a slight edge on keenness of taste).

Most likely you are fat because you equate taste pleasure with high-calory foods (again, a holdover from childhood, when your parents rewarded you with high-calory foods, and when there was no easy access to the large variety of low-calory foods that exists today).

Today there are more delicious low-calory foods, both fresh and frozen, than have ever been in the world's markets. You can have almost any kind of food without being limited to season. You can learn to choose, prepare, and present it so it will be even more appealing to your senses than your former choices. Let's consider the five senses, one by one.

Don't underestimate eye appeal

You're walking down the street. Nothing could be further from your mind than food.

And then you pass a delicatessen. Its windows are filled with fresh onion rolls and doughnuts, plus a creamy cheesecake topped with strawberries in a luxurious, sugary syrup. You walk a little further and you see a billboard advertising spaghetti—a huge plateful of the stuff, dripping with tomato sauce. Your hands start to tremble. Your stomach begs for a treat.

Don't let your eyes fool you. You weren't hungry, remember? This isn't stomach hunger, it's eye hunger.

Conjure up the beautiful thin foods. Picture in your mind's eye a lean, broiled steak, a crisp, cool salad with a delicious low-calorie dressing, a zesty shrimp cocktail.

Remember, too—you're walking down the street. *You* are appealing, because you're thin. Take another look in that delicatessen window—not at the food but at your reflection. Are *you* appealing to look at? Then you're thinking thin.

Your nose is your friend

You walk into a restaurant. A host of aromas floats into your nostrils. Learn to recognize them—learn to pick out the "slim smells." Think of the slim smells and you'll be glad you've got a nose. A leg of lamb spiced with garlic and garnished with mint; a filet of sole accented with lemon and parsley; a juicy slice of rare roast beef with a touch of horse-radish or mustard; a fresh fruit cocktail for dessert. Don't be afraid of your nose.

Give your taste buds a treat

"But my tongue!" you cry in anguish. "My tongue loves to taste strawberry shortcake! My tongue loves to taste spa-ghetti or baked potatoes smothered with sour cream.

Does it really? Wouldn't your tongue be just as happy with strawberries plain? Do you really need all that whipped cream and pastry? Do without it. Savor the strawberries for themselves. Eat as many as you like—they're low in calories and high in vitamins and minerals your body must have to form the enzymes that eat up fat and release energy.

And what about that spaghetti? How much of it does your tongue really taste? Why not settle for a low-calory "meatballs with tomato sauce" dish? Or a crisp, nutritious plate of shrimp or crabmeat with a spicy tomato cocktail sauce that brings out the flavor of the fish rather than dis-guising the lack of flavor in the spaghetti?

That baked potato—yes, you can have a baked potato now and then. But don't double or triple the calories by smearing it with butter or sour cream. Use my low-calory butter or low-calory sour cream—or my "onyurt," a tangy mixture of yogurt and onion powder that is high in protein and low in calories, and perfect with baked potatoes.

Don't smother and drown your taste buds with grease and carbohydrates. *Stimulate them* . . . the natural way.

The textures your teeth love to touch

A great part of the pleasure of eating is the texture of the food. We use words like smooth, creamy, crisp, fine, and coarse to describe texture.

I remember trying to overcome a prejudice against tripe, which is the stomach of an animal.

One day I saw tripe on the menu of one of my favorite Italian restaurants. I ordered it, thinking the taste might be sufficiently disguised in sauce so that I could get it down. It's fun to experiment with new kinds of food.

To my surprise, the sauce was good and the tripe had practically no taste at all—but lots of texture. I did not like eating what seemed to me to be little pieces of sponge. (I still don't.) I asked myself why so many people think so highly of this dish—and then I realized they had developed a *liking* for the texture.

Low-calory foods come in every kind of texture—the creaminess of cottage cheese, the smoothness of meat and and fish, the crispness of vegetables and fruit, the coarseness of salad greens.

Be conscious of the textures of foods. If a particular texture appeals to you, emphasize that texture when selecting low-calory foods.

Snap, crackle, pop

The advertisers of breakfast foods realize so well that the sense of hearing is important in adding pleasure to eating that the words "Snap, Crackle, Pop" have been popularized to indicate fresh, crispy, crunchy cereal. Don't overlook *the sound* of food when looking for the thin foods. Think of fresh, crisp celery sticks, carrots, cucumbers, apples—to mention just a few of the many musical snacks listed later in this book.

Put them together—and you're a sensuous dieter

Encourage your senses to become more aware of the tastiness of low-calory foods. They will be your greatest help in weight reduction. You should be—and probably are—aware of what kind of an eater you are.

Do you prefer to nibble through the day on small, high-calory foods such as cheese and cookies and candy—or do you do your big eating from late afternoon until midnight?

You may, if you are at work, have a stack of candy bars, cheese crackers, and peanut snacks through the early part of the day and move on to serious eating at night. If you are at home all day, you have constant access to all sorts of nibbling.

Whatever your particular weakness, arm yourself with the right kind of ammunition to fight fat. There are many low-calory candies on the market now. These are tasty. They may contain no nutrients at all—but your teeth will be in better condition and you will be thinner if you use them rather than "real" candy. There are also low-calory crackers on the market that are very good. Don't deprive yourself of everything. Don't make a martyr of yourself.

But gradually try to wean yourself from the artificial snacks. At home switch to celery and carrot sticks, radishes, sliced cucumbers, cherry tomatoes, lean cold cuts.

At the office set in a supply of low-calory bouillon cubes. With a portable water heater you can make a surprising variety of nutritious, slimming hot drinks. Thin slices of roast beef or chicken and hard-boiled eggs can be carried from the home to the office and nibbled on throughout the day without noise, mess, or spoilage. More ideas for between-meal snacks are given in Chapter 8.

Don't gorge at any time

The truly sensuous dieter never eats a single mouthful more than what satisfies him. If he does, he is not a sensuous dieter but a glutton.

No matter what your parents told you years ago about cleaning up your plate (reminding you of the starving Armenians, or telling you that you were feeding the devil and starving God), ignore their advice. You will not put one ounce of fat on an Armenian, nor will you please God, if you eat one more mouthful than you want. But you will put more weight on yourself.

Waste not, want not

Don't pile up your plate—or let anyone else do it. Take a longer time to chew your food—you'll have a longer time to experience the pleasurable sensation of taste and texture, and therefore will be satisfied with smaller portions very quickly.

If you are still hungry and have eaten everything on your plate, take a little more. After all, you are now eating only low-calory foods.

In a short time the smaller portions will satisfy you.

Staying Slim the Natural Way does not attempt to analyse *your* reasons for being overweight. Its purpose is to show you how to get slim and stay slim naturally, regardless of why you are fat—and how to enjoy every minute of the new lease on life slimming gives you.

5   Diet Safety

HAVE NO FEAR of losing weight because you think that you will become undernourished. The greatest danger to the health of the American people is overweight. Far more illnesses are caused by being overfed than underfed. Despite stubborn pockets of poverty in many areas, this is the most overfed nation in the world.

You are almost certainly wrong if you think that your overweight is due to glandular imbalance. That is another myth cherished by people who don't want to do anything about losing weight. The percentage of people whose fat is due to glandular malfunction is so small as not to be worth considering here.

Of course you should have regular health checkups, and if you think there is something wrong with the functioning of your glands, you should be under a doctor's care. Ninety-nine times out of a hundred, your doctor will tell you that your fat is due to overeating high-calory foods.

As far as diet safety and pregnancy are concerned (according to a study made by Dr. Istvan Nyirjesy of Georgetown University Medical Center, Washington D.C.), women who are of average weight before becoming pregnant have a better chance of having a baby that will not be stillborn or die shortly after birth than do women who are overweight.

What about cholesterol?

The relationship between fat and the development of hardening of the arteries was first noted many years ago, but the pros and cons of cholesterol and saturated and polyunsaturated fats are still being debated. Saturated fats are mostly found in dairy products and meat. They are solid or almost solid at room temperature.

Many doctors believe that saturated fats accumulate in the arteries, thereby narrowing them, leading to heart attack. These doctors generally recommend the use of polyunsaturated fats for their patients. Polyunsaturated fats are mostly vegetable fats and are liquid at room temperature.

The American Heart Association does not feel that they yet have the complete answer to this question, but they *do* say that there is a real connection between overweight and heart attacks. (For a detailed analysis of this problem, see BOOKS 2000's *Living With Your Heart.*)

Butter vs. margarine

Remember this: There are about the same number of calories in animal fat as in vegetable fat. Many people think that they are taking in fewer calories by using only polyunsaturated fats. This is not true. You are getting *the same number of calories* in each, spoon for spoon. Safflower oil has as many calories as bacon grease; margarine has just about as many calories as butter.

So whether you care about the kind of fat you eat or not, remember that since there are twice as many calories in an ounce of fat as in an ounce of protein or carbohydrates, you will be helping your weight loss greatly if you cut out, or cut down, on foods with visible fat, or those you know have a high fat content.

What about diet pills?

Diet pills may not be harmful if your doctor recommends them, but they should *never* be taken without his supervision. *I do not recommend them!* They are a drug. An overweight person tends to depend on the drug to keep him from being hungry. By having a diet pill he can and often does say to himself, "Okay, pill, now keep me from being hungry. It's up to you!"

It is much better to develop a positive interest in and a liking and desire for low-calory food.

The diet "DT's"

People who are in the habit of eating excessively sometimes get what amounts to withdrawal symptoms when they first start to reduce. Occasionally they complain of headaches, a faint dizziness, nervousness, or slight nausea. This is more psychological than physical and happens because you are changing your habit patterns.

Stick to your guns. If you *really* feel weak, take a spoonful of honey or an ounce of orange juice. The feeling will soon pass away.

Above all, don't worry that you are not getting a balanced diet on low-calory foods. The lists of low calory foods recommended in this book are *nourishing as well as delicious.* When you are in the habit of eating fairly low-fat and low-calory foods and are suddenly confronted with a very rich meal it will often make you sick enough to vomit.

Right after World War II, when our soldiers opened the prison camps to release the prisoners, they brought all kinds of rich foods with them, including pounds of butter (which had been completely absent from the prisoners' diets for months or years). The soldiers thought that they were being good to these deprived people and gave the rich food to them freely. The result of this kindness was a group of terribly sick people. They bloated horribly and more died from this abrupt excess of food than had died from actual malnutrition during the whole period of the existence of the prison camp. It was a sad lesson learned by our armed forces. It is harder to accommodate our systems to overfeeding than underfeeding.

A word about "store-bought" low-calory foods

Your local supermarket probably has a special section devoted to low-calory or dietetic foods. Here you'll find salad dressings of all kinds, mayonnaise, jellies and jams, canned fruits and vegetables—new products every time you look.

Read the labels carefully. Some of them may be misleading. Is that low-calory mayonnaise really low-calory? Or is it just "polyunsaturated"? On a recent trip to my market I discovered some unpleasant surprises among several happy ones. The so-called low-calory mayonnaise wasn't low-calory. The label proclaimed, in small type, that one tablespoon contained 100 calories—the same as ordinary mayonnaise. The only thing "dietetic" about it was that it used safflower oil instead of olive oil!

Many of these products also state clearly on their labels: "To be used only by persons who must restrict their intake of sugar." Well, if you're going to lose weight you *must* restrict your intake of sugar. But don't get hooked on these products when you can make your own at home and know exactly what's going into them. The chemicals listed in the ingredients are sometimes enough to make a pharmacist blanch.

Also, don't stick just to the diet section. Low-calory foods can be found elsewhere in your market. A recent inspection of cottage cheese revealed that of three brands—two "1-per-

cent fat" cottage cheeses, one skim-milk cottage cheese—
each had a different amount of calories per tablespoon. Read
the labels and choose the one with the lowest.

Go to the soft-drink section and you'll find a number of
low-calory refreshers that do not contain cyclamates. Again
you will find the warning on the label. Don't let it frighten
you. Low-calory soft drinks, taken in moderation, are a
wonderful way of getting a nice, full feeling in your stomach.

Remember that margarine has as many calories as butter,
and that low-calory margarine is usually only regular margarine mixed with water and blown up with air. You might
as well buy regular margarine, add a little water, and whip
it up in the blender. It's cheaper. Cheaper still, my low-calory
butter (see page 58).

You'll also find low-calory, high-protein breads and thinly
sliced bread, and high-protein spaghetti and macaroni. There
are calories here, but if you must have spaghetti (and you
may, occasionally), buy the high-protein variety.

When you are looking for tuna fish, salmon, crab meat, or
sardines, look for the fish that is packed in water, not oil. In
short, keep your eyes open and read the labels.

Again, read the labels. A recent survey of "diet" drinks
showed one to have 0.6 calories per ounce, another to have
3.5 calories per ounce, and a third to have 6.5 calories per
ounce! All three are still much lower in calories than their
nondiet counterparts.

What about salt?

It is true that salt has no calories. It is also true that salt
retains fluids in your body—fluids that you want to get rid of
to lose weight. However, unless you have a passion for salt,
or your doctor prescribes a low sodium diet, it is not necessary for you to be overly concerned about it.

As far as your body's need for salt: there are times when you perspire greatly and may need a little extra salt—take a tablet or a teaspoonful without fear.

What About Sugar?

Sugar has no food value to speak of, and it does have considerable calories. Still, it is a quick source of energy and it does make food taste sweet. You must learn to reduce your intake of sugar. Substitute saccharine or switch to foods that are naturally sweet. Many people including myself sweeten foods and beverages with honey or maple syrup. This is an excellent idea, for honey and maple syrup are rich in vitamins and minerals . . . but don't be misled: *They have just as many calories as sugar.*

6 Exercise Can Be Easy

UNLESS YOU ARE a Hollywood sex goddess, your face is the one part of your body most frequently recalled by your friends. It is what strikes them most quickly as looking good, younger, or older.

Yet in any exercise program the face is almost always the one neglected body part. At the same time, it is the face that many of us blame for not sticking to a good weight-control program.

Many carboholics give this excuse for staying fat:

"Whenever I lose a few pounds my skin gets so droopy and flabby, and I look so awful, I decide to start eating. I may be fat, but at least my skin is firm."

Don't believe a word of it. It's natural to be slim. If you lose weight naturally there's no reason for your face or skin to sag or droop.

It is true that occasionally, when a *huge amount of fast weight loss occurs,* the skin's elasticity does not rebound as quickly as the fat is lost, and it may take a short while after the big loss for you to regain that firm, young look.

But if you persevere with viewing food in a new way, selecting low-calory foods for their deliciousness as well as their low calory content and high nutrient content, you will lose weight— and your skin will never suffer.

But what about aging?

As we get older our faces, like every other part of our bodies, undergo certain changes. To what extent these changes make us look more or less attractive *can* be determined by us, to some degree. We can also delay—and even prevent—some of the changes.

First let's look at the skin itself. What can you do to keep it clear and wrinkle-free?

Massaging your face with creams will help—but only if such massaging makes you feel better! Nothing improves the looks of a face quite as much as a pair of sparkling eyes and a cheerful smile. If you have a reasonably uncomplicated personal life, if you maintain your ideal weight level by eating nutritious foods, your skin will be smooth and clear—provided it gets enough moisture.

There are literally hundreds of so-called beauty creams on the market today that claim to preserve the texture of the skin. You can easily spend hundreds of dollars a year on the more expensive of these creams.

Now the creams are not going to hurt you (unless you are allergic to one or more of the chemicals in them). But neither will they make a significant contribution to your skin.

The natural—and only—way to preserve skin is to feed it from within by getting nourishing food, and to protect it on the outside by avoiding sun and giving your skin moisture.

A coating of facial cream will keep some moisture in; a more efficient and less expensive treatment is to get a room moisturizer. During the winter months our homes are too often overheated and moistureless. Our skin dries out. It loses moisture. It does not lose oil.

And so you apply cream—and the cream *does* form a thin layer over your face and tends to slow the dehydration.

It would be of far greater help to your skin and your respiratory system if, instead of buying expensive creams, you would save your money and buy one or more humidifiers to put moisture back in your house during the winter months.

The humidity in a room is ideal if a humidity gauge registers 35 to 55. (A humidity gauge is inexpensive and should be checked with the regularity that you check the thermometer on your thermostat.)

In the summer there is often the problem of too *much* humidity in the air: This causes discomfort but is not harmful to your skin. What *is* harmful is the sun. You are not a lizard and it is not natural for you, as it is for him, to lie out in the sun and bake. If you insist on it, you will soon begin to look like a lizard.

Danger from the sun

Not only does the heat from the sun dry out the moisture in your skin; the sun's rays cause premature aging (not to mention skin cancer).

Avoid the sun like the plague if you want your skin to retain its soft, youthful texture. If you must go out into it (for gardening, swimming, and other sports) the best protection is a liquid or cream that filters out the rays, plus an opaque-colored makeup base. Sun hats and umbrellas are also helpful (I have a redheaded friend who takes his umbrella into the pool with him).

Aside from protecting you from the sun, creams are best for removing makeup. The perfect beauty treatment—and the natural one—is a thorough washing with very mild soap, rinsing well with *soft* water, and staying in a properly humidified atmosphere.

Even the clearest, most lustrous skin holds little attraction to the beholder when it covers saggy, flabby facial muscles.

Yes, your face has muscles, and when you look into the mirror at jowls, dewlaps, double chins you are not looking at sagging skin but at sagging muscles and at fat.

It is a wonder that men, who are otherwise rather vain of their physique, never seem to pay much attention to the musculature of their faces.

Perhaps they never realized that they actually have muscles in their faces and heads. Or perhaps they have just felt that there is nothing to be done about the aging process in the face.

Women spend a great deal of time and money on their faces—but again neglect the muscles of the face.

The value of facial exercise

When you grow older there is a loss in the fatty layer beneath the skin on your face. If you have good tonus in the musculature underneath, you can retard the aging process (wrinkling and sagging) for a long time.

To have good tonus in the muscles anywhere in the body, the tissues must be well nourished and the muscles must get exercise. We all talk more or less throughout the day and thus do get some facial exercise. But we tend to overexercise part of our faces and underexercise the rest, leaving the tonus in our faces unbalanced. This imbalance more often accounts for change in the appearance of the face than aging from wrinkling does.

There are a few simple exercises for the face and neck that will do wonders to keep it from ever really sagging.

You can do these exercises any time of the day, in just a few minutes. You are more apt to do them regularly, and benefit from them, if you incorporate them into your early-morning ritual while you are looking into the mirror, just before or after shaving or applying makeup. At one point in my life I did these exercises while driving to work, in Chicago. As I sped along the Loop sticking out my tongue, wrinkling my nose, shaking my head, and blowing out my cheeks, I'm afraid I rather startled a good many fellow commuters. But I kept my tonus up.

Five easy face fixer-uppers

(1) Hold your index finger against your lips, as if you were signaling *hush*. Blow your cheeks out, pushing your index finger hard against your lips to keep air from escaping. Count up to six to yourself while blowing out your cheeks. Doing this exercise ten times will firm up your cheeks.

(2) Purse your lips as for whistling; while keeping them in that position try to wrinkle up your nose. You will feel the tension of the muscles along the sides of the nose if you hold the whistle position of the lips while wrinkling. Repeat 10 times. This exercise helps to erase the lines at the sides of the cheeks near the nose.

(3) Stick out your tongue as far as you can, arching it as high as you can while you do so. If you place your index and third finger under your chin, back close to your neck you will be able to feel the tension in the muscle. This exercise is unbeatable for keeping a firm chin line. Do it 10 times.

(4) Close your eyes and look up toward the ceiling. Count five while you hold them in this position. Do this 10 times. Now close them again and look down, again holding them in this position. Do this 10 times. You can do the eye exercises without closing your eyes, but this tends to wrinkle the forehead. If you touch the area just beneath the eye while you are doing the first part of this exercise you will feel the tension in the muscle there. You will feel the same with the

second part of the exercise if you touch your eyelid while you are doing it.

This exercise prevents bags from forming under the eyes, and also helps to relax and rest them too.

(5) The muscles in the neck respond so quickly to a little exercise, and firmness in the neck improves your appearance tremendously.

Interlace your fingers and place the interlaced palm sides against your forehead. While you count up to five, push against your hands with your head at the same time that you are trying to push your head back with the interlaced palms of your hands.

Now place the interlaced fingers at the back of your head, palm sides against your hair. Push and resist, counting up to five.

Now place the palm of your right hand against the right side of your head, against the hair, just behind your temple and just above the ear. Push and resist, counting up to five. Do the same with the left hand on the left side of the head.

What About Gelatin?

Periodically the women of America go on a gelatin kick, imagining that drinking a solution of the stuff will work all sorts of miraculous cures—relax them, put them to sleep, cure dandruff and baldness, and most popularly, give them stronger fingernails.

There is no scientific evidence to support any of this. But gelatin does remain a low-calory, high-protein product that is useful in making all kinds of delicious, low-calory desserts and salads.

No time for your body

Although the need to exercise your body is less strange to you than the need to exercise your face, if you are like most people you either cannot or do not wish to stay on an organized program of exercise. *Such a program is not necessary to the maintenance of flexibility and good muscle tone.*

Whether you engage actively and regularly in some sport, or whether you like to take walks for exercise, or even if you dislike any more exercise than is necessary to get from one place to another, the important thing is to *make your movements count for the beauty of your body.*

When man picked himself up from all fours, he put the kind of stress on his body that has brought him all sorts of aches and pains. In order to combat this upright position's weakness it is necessary to get the most help from the frame (which is the skeleton of the body) by using it to carry as much balanced weight as possible.

The minimum of movement, done correctly, will mean more health to your muscles than working out all day without correct body alignment.

The upright human back should be straight. This is easier said than done, since few of us know what a really straight back is. The simplest way of aligning your body is to stand with your back pressed against a straight wall. Feel your spine touch the wall. Feel your body touch the wall from the back of your head (your head held straight with chin slightly in), all the way down your back, pelvis pushed under, legs and knees straight down to your heels.

This position is not too easy to achieve right away, since most people do not keep their pelvis tucked under with knees and legs held straight.

In the anthropological section of a Paris museum, there is

a remarkable exhibit. It's a photograph of a Hottentot woman, taken in life, along with a death cast of her body—plus her actual skeleton. She had been a mistress of a French marquis, who apparently considered her anatomy worthy of immortality. He must have had a bizarre taste: The exhibit shows how dreadfully the body can be deliberately distorted. The woman's whole pelvic region had been bent back to make her buttocks appear as if they were a shelf. If ever the barbaric fashion of an exaggerated rear becomes stylish again (at it was in the 1880's, when it was à la mode to wear the bustle, carried on the back of the gown, below a well-corseted waist), I do hope that the ladies will relegate the fashion to dress ornamentation only, and firmly reject the body-distorting corset.

If you get the idea of a straight back fixed in your consciousness, there are many times through the day that you will be reminded to straighten out. Doing this will be a rest for your back.

When you go up to the tee before you take your stance for a golf swing, straighten out, then take your stance.

When you are before the net in a tennis match, before you start playing, straighten out. Do so again during the rest period. It will rest your body greatly if you stretch up with your hands and arms reaching toward the sky, head level on your shoulders.

If you have difficulty feeling your spine touch all the way when you press your back against a straight wall, try doing it in bed at night or when you first wake up in the morning. Stretch out flat on your back without a pillow and you will have better luck attaining this straight position. Stretch your body long—with feet turned up toward the ceiling. Feel as if you are pushing your heels toward the bottom of the bed . . .

suck in your abdomen . . . feel your spine make contact with the bed all along your back.

It is a marvelous sensation. While you are in this position try to become aware of how your whole body feels. Picture yourself walking with your back this straight, and as you walk *lift your knees instead of shuffling your feet,* and kick your feet out from the knees. When you get out of bed try to repeat this feeling as you actually walk.

You will be getting more correct exercise than you have had for years. *If you just stood up against the wall for three to five minutes a day, flattening your spine against it, you could throw out all other exercise.*

During the course of a day, when you bend, either bend at the hips, keeping the back and knees straight, or keep the back straight and just bend the knees and balance on the toes. It doesn't take more time to do this, just more thought— and you will be giving yourself a great workout.

When you are near the kitchen or bathroom sink, step back from it (about a foot and a half at first, then later increase the distance) and stretch your arms out, leaning against the sink with your abdomen sucked in and your knees straight. Keep your body (your back) straight, bend your elbows, letting your body go in toward the sink as in a push-up. Then straighten your elbows, pushing your body back to an upright position.

Exercise Machines

Forget belts, straps, and all kinds of gimmicks and machines to tone your muscles. At best they are worthless and some have been proven to be very dangerous to use. It is the natural way that will bring results.

For men only

One great way for a man to stretch the tendons and muscles in the back of the legs without killing him (since he is almost always tighter there than a woman) is to bend over at the hips and just hang for a minute or two. He will find that if he relaxes in this position his body will slowly start stretching out by itself. Come back from this position slowly because coming up fast will let the muscles and tendons snap back too fast.

In a few days you will be greatly surprised at how much closer to the floor your hands will go without trying.

The above exercises may seem too easy to amount to anything because they don't hurt. And they are easy . . . because they're natural.

If you really try to keep this straight body in mind during all the movements you make through the day you will have a fabulous exercise program without changing your way of life.

It takes a little prodding to keep this position in mind as as you walk around. It takes no extra movement. It only takes a little thought to pick up your feet by lifting your knees slightly, keeping your abdomen in and your back straight.

It is really a wonder why anyone stands the discomfort of the muscles that comes from years of distorted posture.

And never forget that exercising can be romantic, too. Dancing is a superb exercise. If you aren't in a position to get out to nightclubs regularly, dance at home—to a lively television commercial, do a few exotic ballet steps (invent them yourself) along with Dean Martin or Glen Campbell. Even lovemaking is good exercise; passionate kissing is marvelous exercise for the muscles of the face.

7 Eating Your Way to a Thin You

NOW THAT YOU KNOW THE MAJOR CAUSES of overweight and the dangers involved in being overweight, and have learned a few easy exercises to keep your muscles firm, you must learn just what are the natural, thin foods. How can you prepare them in exciting and tasty ways? How can you adapt these foods to your daily life—when dining at home, when dining at a restaurant, when visiting a friend?

First you will need to establish a regular pattern of eating. Here are two menus to work with. One is an *ideal menu*. The other is a menu tailored to our modern day life.

Under ideal conditions you should eat a large breakfast, a hearty lunch, and a light dinner. But many of us simply don't have time or appetite for a large breakfast. At lunch we are forced to grab a quick sandwich. And at dinnertime the whole family is together, we entertain, and we want to have that large meal that we don't really need at the end of the day.

Try to adapt the ideal menu to your life-style. If you can't, work from the secondary menu, making such improvisations and variations as you wish.

IDEAL MENU

Breakfast

One slice of whole wheat toast, buttered with my low-calory butter.

Three to four ounces of lean broiled meat (pork chop, ham, lamb chop, liver; avoid bacon).

Fresh fruit: One-half grapefruit or one orange. *Or* stewed prunes or apricots. *Or* one glass of fruit juice.

One glass skim milk.

Hot beverage, if desired (coffee or tea, without milk or sugar).

Note: Eggs are traditional breakfast fare, and many of us cannot conceive of a breakfast without them. However, the yolks are high in cholesterol, and many heart specialists warn against having more than three eggs a week.

If you want to substitute eggs for meat, be sure to cook them without fat—boiled, poached, or scrambled in a non-stick pan.

Midmorning Snack

Choose from my list of snacks for sneak eaters, p. 54

Lunch

Tossed green salad with one of my low-calory dressings.
One cooked green vegetable.

Three to four ounces of lean meat, broiled (or choose from my list of entrees).

One glass of skim milk.

Fresh fruit (or choose from my list of desserts).

Afternoon Snack

Choose from my list of low-calory snacks for sneak eaters.

Cocktail Hour

See "Lose with Booze" p. 87.

Dinner

One bowl of soup, *or* Tossed green salad.

Fresh fruit and cheese. *Or* choose from my list of low-calory desserts.

Bedtime Snack

One 6-ounce glass of skim milk.

One slice of whole wheat toast or two dietetic cookies (or choose from my low-calory snacks for sneak eaters).

SECOND-BEST MENU

Breakfast

One glass of orange juice.

One egg (see above for preparation).

One slice of whole wheat toast.

One hot beverage, without sugar or cream

Midmorning Snack

Same as in ideal menu.

Lunch

One bowl of low-calory soup.

One slice of whole wheat bread.

One tossed salad *or*

One sandwich made with unbuttered whole wheat or rye bread, thinly sliced. Use lettuce, lean, thinly sliced meat, or a meat salad (chicken, ham, shrimp, tuna, etc.) made with my low-calory mayonnaise. Served with glass skim milk.

Fresh fruit or yogurt, flavored or plain.

Midafternoon Snack

Same as in ideal menu.

Cocktail hour

Same as in ideal menu.

Dinner

Three to four ounces of lean meat, broiled (or one of my entrees).

One cooked green vegetable, seasoned with lemon juice, broth, or my low-calory salad dressings.

One tossed green salad.

Fresh fruit or one of my low-calory desserts.

Nighttime Snack

One cup hot bouillon and one of my low-calory snacks for sneak eaters.

or

One 6-ounce glass of skim milk.

Note: You may drink all the coffee and tea you want (no sugar or cream) but remember that both drinks have no vitamins but lots of caffein.

Stocking the low-calory larder

Earlier in this book I told you that there are, today, hundreds of exciting new products that make low-calory cooking more imaginative and easier than ever. Now I'm going to tell you about them in detail.

First there are certain basic staples that you should have on hand at all times. These foods are easy to find and inexpensive. Here's a suggested starter larder:

6 cans of chicken broth
6 cans of beef broth
2 jars of chicken bouillon cubes
2 jars of beef bouillon cubes
4 cans of tomato bisque
4 cans of vegetable juice (V8)
4 cans of tomato juice
4 cans of evaporated skim milk
2 jars of onion powder
1 jar of celery powder
1 jar of dry dill weed
1 jar of oregano
1 jar of ground cumin seed
1 jar cayenne pepper
1 jar of powdered cinnamon
1 jar of ginger
1 jar of paprika
1 jar of nutmeg
Whole black pepper, to grind
2 small bottles of vanilla extract
2 small bottles of imitation butter flavoring
1 small bottle each of orange, lemon, banana, strawberry and raspberry flavoring
1 jar yellow food coloring
1 jar liquid saccharin
Your favorite herbs and spices

Let me now give you an explanation for some of the more unusual items on the list.

Broth is beautiful

Once you're on the road to gourmet, low-calorie dining, you're going to use enormous quantities of broth. All of your soups will use broth.

Yes, you can make your own broth by boiling down bones and vegetable trimmings. I used to make my own broth (recipes for homemade broth can be found in any standard cookbook).

I don't anymore. I just don't have the time for the long hours of gentle simmering, skimming off the fat, and clarifying the liquid.

Canned broth is delicious and economical. Refrigerate

canned chicken broth before using. A small amount of fat will congeal on the surface and can easily be scraped off with a teaspoon.

Bouillon cubes dissolve in hot water in seconds. Gourmet hint: don't add extra salt when using the cubes.

Miracle milk

Today most of the companies that manufacture evaporated milk also manufacture *evaporated skim milk*. If your local supermarket does not yet carry it, make sure it does. This wonderful, fat-free milk is rich and creamy. You'll be using it to make your own butter, your own mayonnaise, your own hollandaise, and dozens and dozens of creamy, fat-free soups.

Onions and celery

The French add onions and celery to practically every meat and fish dish they make. You should, too—but you needn't waste time peeling and chopping and weeping.

I believe that the flavor of onion improves everything except dessert—and you may even know a dessert that would be improved by it. Today I use onion powder almost to the exclusion of fresh onion; it is real onion and has a true onion flavor. (I don't recommend garlic powder because to me it has an off or preserved taste. If you like garlic, use it fresh. Onion powder, incidentally, is different from onion flakes and minced onion, which do not lend themselves so easily to so many recipes.)

With onion powder you avoid smelly fingers and the extra calories that come when you must fry the onions in butter or oil. You can brown onion powder in your frying pan without using any oil at all.

Celery powder, sometimes called ground celery seed, is

another all-purpose ingredient that adds a special flavoring to every food. Don't confuse it with celery salt, which I see no excuse for. Two other new low-calory products for gourmet flavors: shallot powder and mushroom powder.

Utensils for space-age kitchens

There are certain utensils that you really ought to have to make your kitchen tasks easy and fun. Some of them are not cheap. But when you consider the money they save you in expensive, fatty ingredients, the time they save you, the saved hospital bills, the cost is incidental. If you don't already have them, start saving for them, and drop broad hints at Christmas, birthday, or anniversary.

The blender

Fortunately the blender has been around for a long time, and most people have one. It's indispensible for making my low-calory butter, sour cream, and the various sauces and salad dressings. Put this first on your list.

Nonstick skillets and saucepans

One of the great cooking discoveries of this or any century: ideal for frying meat, fish, and eggs without oil or butter.

Double boiler

For slow, nutritious cooking and scrambling eggs without oil or butter.

Broiling pan with rack

From now on you're going to broil or roast most of your meat and fish in the oven. The meat will sit on the rack: The fat will drip off it into the pan below. Try it with a chicken. Don't dip the chicken in anything. Just rinse it, dry it, place it on the rack, and pop it into a 375° oven for an hour or an hour and a half (depending on its size). Fifteen minutes before taking it out of the oven sprinkle a little paprika over the breast, thighs, and legs.

When you serve it, it will be a glorious brown, with a crisp, crunchy, delicious skin.

For gravy, pour off the fat in the pan, add a little water and lemon juice, and bring to a boil on your range, stirring constantly to mix in the chicken juices—a lovely, golden, low-calorie gravy. Use the same technique for all kinds of roasts, steak, fish filets, ribs, etc. (Oven temperature and time of cooking naturally vary with the nature of the meat.)

Portable, open-hearth oven

One of the oldest methods of cooking, this is also the most modern. There are several kinds of portable open-hearth ovens on the market today, most of them with rotisserie attachments. They range in price from $20 to $200 and provide you with the most nutritious and delicious—and easy—methods of cooking meat and fish imaginable. A booklet of instructions and recipes is usually included in the box.

Pepper mill

For the delicious taste of freshly ground pepper.

The home freezer

Although a major investment—and often impractical for apartment dwellers—the home freezer can help keep you slim and healthy in a variety of ways:

- Leftover bread, rolls, cakes, casseroles, etc. should be frozen rather than stored in the refrigerator; in the freezer they are out of reach and out of mind. You will not be able to nibble on them throughout the day, and will think twice before thawing them. Resist temptation by freezing it.

- A number of delicious low-calory desserts (sherbets, mousse, my ice creams) require freezing. See my recipes, p. 78.

- If you shop for a week or so in advance, freezing various meats, fish, and vegetables that you do not plan to eat within a day or two preserves nutrients and retards spoilage. One good general rule to remember: The less fat a meat has, the longer it will freeze.

You can actually save money with a freezer by stocking up on foods that are on sale—so *do* investigate the possibility of getting a freezer if you do not already have one. There are now low-cost portable freezers on the market that are suitable for most apartment dwellers.

Hints for the low-calory chef

Now you have the basic foods and equipment to get started. Before we get into the recipes let's take a look at some quick tricks that will help you to get maximum flavor and nutrition and minimum calories from the foods you cook.

Meat tenderizers

Commercial meat tenderizers are not recommended for the less tender cuts of meat. When tenderizing is called for it is much better, and much more natural, to marinate the meat. A marinade dressing is made with vinegar or lemon or lime juice and any herb you like. Just cover the less tender cuts of meat with this marinade sauce and let them stand in the refrigerator a few hours or even overnight. This adds flavor as it tenderizes the meat.

Since Americans are big consumers of hamburgers, you and your children will probably continue to be. In order to get the leanest beef for hamburgers, order flank steak and have it ground twice to insure tenderness. It is one of the most *flavorful* parts of beef and is delicious unground and barbecued out of doors, or broiled in your oven broiler if it has been marinated a few hours or overnight before cooking.

Trimming fat

The fat on meat should be trimmed as much as possible before cooking or freezing. When that is impossible (when you are in a restaurant, for example, or in the home of a friend), trim it as you eat it and leave it on your plate. The theory that leaving the fat on the roast adds flavor is nonsense to the low-calorie chef.

Cooking vegetables

Whether you use water or broth for cooking your vegetables (and most are more delicious when cooked in broth, either beef or chicken), *don't drown them in the liquid*. Always use the least amount that will cook them without burning.

If you wish to add a bouillon cube for additional flavor, wait until the vegetable is done and add just enough of it to flavor and salt the vegetable. The bouillon cube is very salty, and salt added to water or stock *before* cooking draws the minerals out of the vegetables into the liquid and leaves them less nourishing—unless you consume every bit of the liquid. When you cook vegetables in broth, additional flavorings such as butter are usually not necessary.

⑧ Recipes for Thin Gourmets

The following recipes, soup through dessert, are low in calories and are all delicious enough to serve for company dinners.

True hunger pangs are caused by contractions in the stomach. These contractions occur when the stomach has been empty for a certain period of time. False hunger pangs occur when you start thinking about fatty foods and begin to feel sorry for yourself.

Whether you are experiencing false hunger pangs or true ones, the quickest way of getting rid of them without eating is to keep your stomach filled with liquids.

The only liquids that have no calories are water, black coffee, and tea (without sugar, milk, or cream). These may fill you, but they have no nutritional value and may over-stimulate you.

Low-calory drinks

There are a number of drinks that are sufficiently low in calories to give you enough variety, satisfaction, and nutrition to warrant drinking them.

Keep a variety of natural juices on hand—tomato, vegetable, orange, sauerkraut, grape, grapefruit, apple, clam, etc. Hot broth made with bouillon cubes is an excellent substitute for coffee. So is hot tomato juice.

You may drink low-calorie soft drinks if you like, but read the label on the can or bottle carefully, and drink them in moderation: Colas contain considerable caffein, and if you think "dieting" makes you nervous and irritable, filling up with caffein is not going to help you.

Club soda plain or flavored with lemon or lime juice is a zesty "adult" drink.

There is another way to avoid fatty snacks; put in a supply of low-calorie snacks that will be tasty and satisfying and will not build up your calorie intake. Here are some suggestions:

Snacks for snack eaters

Meat snacks

Landjaeger (These are small sausages about the size of a small frankfurter—delicious for snacks.)	Salami, German (Hard) Salami, Italian (Hard) Salami, Hungarian (Hard)
Summer Sausage (Hard) Salami, Jewish (Hard)	Dried Beef (The kind that comes in packages: It is less salty than that which comes in jars.)

Keep plenty of vegetable snacks in the refrigerator:

Carrot sticks	Radishes
Celery sticks	Cucumbers
Zucchini slices	Scallions

CHILI CON CARNE (WITHOUT BEANS)

A small bowl of this will be most satisfying.

1 lb flank steak ground twice	*1 tsp ground celery seed*
1 (No. 2) can tomato puree	*1 Tbsp ground cumin*
1 (No. 2) can tomatoes	*¼ to ½ tsp (depending on*
4 Tbsp onion powder	*taste) Cayenne pepper*

Brown the ground meat in a nonstick skillet. Drain off the grease, if any, and add the other ingredients. Simmer 30 minutes.

BASIC BAKED CUSTARD

1½ cups skimmed milk	*1 egg yolk*
2 whole eggs	

Scald milk (just bring it to a boil and turn off the heat). Beat whole eggs and extra yolk together till well mixed, and add scalded milk. (The flavoring for the various custards will have been added to the milk previously.) Pour into individual cups. Set cups in a pan of hot water. Bake in a slow oven 325° for one hour or until inserted knife comes out clean.

CHICKEN CUSTARD

The recipe for Basic Custard (given above). To hot milk, add 2 chicken bouillon cubes.

1 tsp powdered onion	*1 tsp chopped chives*
¼ tsp ground celery seed	*1 cup white meat of chicken,*
1 tsp chopped parsley	*minced.*

Proceed as for Basic Custard, but add the seasonings this time to the hot milk. Just before pouring the egg mixture, divide chicken and chives, put some into each cup, then pour. Bake as above.

CRAB CUSTARD

Make the same as Chicken Custard—using crab meat.

SWEET CUSTARD

Basic Baked Custard recipe
9 *saccharin tablets, or*
3 *Tbsp granulated sugar or brown sugar, or*
3 *Tbsp pure maple syrup, or*

4 *Tbsp honey*
1 *tsp vanilla or 1 tsp orange —or 1 tsp lemon, or 1 tsp raspberry, or 1 tsp of strawberry flavoring*

Add the sweeteners to milk and proceed as with Basic Custard.

HARD-COOKED EGGS IN JELLIED BOUILLON

1 *Tbsp unflavored gelatin*
2 *cups chicken or beef broth (canned)*
4 *hard-cooked eggs*
2 *chicken or beef bouillon cubes*

½ *tsp Dijon mustard*
1 *tsp onion powder*
¼ *tsp ground celery seed*
1 *tsp vinegar*
8 *slices hard salami or summer sausage*

Soften gelatin in ¼ cup of either the chicken or beef broth. Heat the rest of the broth to boiling, add to softened gelatin, and stir until gelatin is dissolved.

Add chicken and beef cubes to this mixture and dissolve them. Set mixture aside to cool.

Cut hard-cooked eggs in halves, lengthwise. Remove the yolks. Mash the salami or summer sausage into very small bits and add to the egg yolks, along with the mustard, vinegar, and celery and onion powder.

Stuff this mixture back into the egg whites. Arrange the stuffed eggs in a dish, cover with the gelatin, and chill in the refrigerator until the gelatin has set.

DRIED BEEF ROLLS

1 cup thick low-calory sour
   cream

2 Tbsp drained horseradish

Mix cream and horseradish thoroughly and spread fairly
thickly on slices of dried beef. Roll up the beef and chill
before serving.

HAM AND ASPARAGUS ROLL

Marinate cooked asparagus in low-calory French dressing.
Drain, roll in thin slices of boiled ham. This makes a delicious
and unusual first course.

STUFFED EGGS

3 hard-boiled eggs
1 Tbsp low-calory French
   dressing

1 tsp onion powder
¼ tsp ground celery seed
¼ cup hard salami, minced

Cut hard-boiled eggs in half, remove yolks, put white aside.
Mash yolks with all other ingredients. Stuff egg-white halves.

MELON MOLD SALAD

1 small melon
1 package lemon, lime, or
   orange gelatin

1 cup boiling water
¾ cup low-calory sour cream

Peel a whole melon. Cut a slice from one end and remove
the seeds. Then drain well and turn upside down. Dissolve
gelatin in boiling water, add cold water and let cool completely. Pour into melon and chill until firm. Slice the melon,
arrange the slices on beds of romaine lettuce or individual
plates or a serving platter, spread thick, low-calory sour cream
over the slices. Chill and serve.

Low-calory gourmet sauces

The low-calory sauces and dressings listed in this chapter are delicious on many different foods. As all good cooks know, many sauces used on salads or dressings can be used on meats with minor differences of flavoring.

French dressing is good on a tossed green salad—everyone knows that. But it's also good on tomatoes, asparagus, broccoli, and even chilled shrimp!

Experiment. You may make a few mistakes, but each mistake will teach you something.

LOW-CALORY BUTTER

I was really tickled when I discovered this easy way to make "butter." It looks like butter . . . tastes like butter . . . and is a wonderful food, low in calories, high in protein and nutrients. Spread it on toast, waffles, pancakes, potatoes, vegetables—and use as much as you like.

1 cup "diet" or skim-milk cottage cheese	*½ tsp butter flavoring (optional)*
¼ cup evaporated skim milk	*¼ tsp yellow food coloring*
	¼ tsp salt

Put the ingredients in the blender and blend until creamy, adding a little more evaporated milk if necessary. Store in the refrigerator. (Not to be used in cooking.)

LOW-CALORY SOUR CREAM

1 cup "diet" or skim-milk cottage cheese	*¼ cup buttermilk*
	1 tsp lemon juice

Put the ingredients in the blender and blend until creamy, adding a little more buttermilk if necessary. Store in the refrigerator.

LOW-CALORY MAYONNAISE

1 cup "diet" or skim-milk
    cottage cheese
¼ cup evaporated skim milk
¼ cup vinegar

½ tsp white pepper
1 tsp onion powder
1 tsp dry mustard
1 tsp celery powder

Put the ingredients in the blender and blend until creamy, adding a little more buttermilk if necessary. Store in the refrigerator. (Not to be used in cooking.)

CUCUMBER SAUCE

A fine sauce for chicken and fish dishes.

1½ cups my low-calory sour
    cream (above)
2 tsp onion powder

¼ tsp ground celery seed
2 cucumbers (peeled)

Put peeled cucumbers in blender and blend fine but don't liquefy. Put in strainer and let stand to let all possible liquid drain off

Now mix the drained pulp with the remaining ingredients. Chill.

HORSERADISH DRESSING

This is good with beef or tongue.

1 cup my low-calory sour
    cream (above)
½ cup drained horseradish

½ tsp onion powder
Pinch of ground celery seed
Salt to taste

Mix all ingredients in blender. Chill.

ONYURT

1 cup plain yogurt
1 tsp onion powder

¼ tsp celery powder

Stir well, adding more onion powder for a stronger taste.

MUSTARD SAUCE

This is good with fish, meat, or vegetables, hot or cold.

1 tsp tarragon vinegar	2 tsp onion powder
1 tsp malt vinegar	¼ tsp ground celery seed
1 tsp cider vinegar	1 Tbsp vegetable oil
1 Tbsp Dijon mustard	2 hard-cooked egg yolks

Blend thoroughly in blender.

LOW-CALORY FRENCH DRESSING (BASIC)

¼ cup lemon juice	½ tsp marjoram
¼ cup tarragon vinegar	½ tsp dill weed
¼ cup wine vinegar	½ tsp salt
1 tsp powdered onion	2 Tbsp boiled water
¼ tsp ground celery seed	2 Tbsp vegetable oil

Mix all of the above ingredients, adding the oil last. To the above Basic French Dressing, you can add chopped hard-boiled eggs, garlic, other herbs, or 1 tablespoon chili sauce.

BLUE CHEESE DRESSING

¼ cup blue cheese	¼ cup my low-calory French dressing
¼ cup my low-calory sour cream, or	

Crush the cheese with a fork and stir in either my sour cream (above) or French dressing.

THOUSAND ISLAND DRESSING

½ cup my low-calory sour cream (above), or	½ cup yogurt
	2 Tbsp barbecue sauce

Stir the barbecue sauce into the sour cream or the yogurt, adding additional barbecue sauce for a stronger flavor.

GREEN GODDESS DRESSING

1 clove garlic, crushed
3 Tbsp anchovy paste
3 Tbsp finely snipped chives

⅓ cup finely snipped parsley
1 cup of my low-calory
    mayonnaise (above)

Mix all ingredients. Cover and chill. Salt and pepper to taste.

LEMON SAUCE

This gourmet sauce goes well with fish, lamb, and chicken.

1½ cup chicken broth
1 chicken bouillon cube
1 Tbsp grated lemon peel
Juice of ½ lemon

2 tsp cornstarch
½ tsp onion powder
¼ tsp ground celery seed

Mix a little of the broth with cornstarch; mix until very smooth. Add the rest of the broth slowly, then all the rest of the ingredients. Cook over low heat, stirring constantly, until mixture starts to thicken. Remove from heat.

CREOLE SAUCE

1 Tbsp onion powder
¼ tsp ground celery seed
⅓ cup green pepper, chopped
    fine
⅓ cup mushroom chopped
    fine (but not as fine
    as peppers)

⅓ cup stuffed green olives
½ chicken bouillon cube
½ beef bouillon cube
1½ cups canned tomatoes

Brown powdered onion and ground celery seed in pan (no fat needed). Keep stirring so it does not burn. Add the rest of the ingredients and let it simmer about ten minutes, until it cooks down and has thickened a little. Fine with fish, chicken or eggs.

EGG SAUCE

1 can evaporated skimmed
   milk
2 raw eggs
2 hard-cooked egg yolks,
   chopped fine

1 tsp onion powder
½ tsp ground celery seed
¼ cup chicken broth
1 chicken bouillon cube

Heat chicken broth. Dissolve bouillon cube in the broth and put aside to cool. Beat raw egg yolks and stir the evaporated milk into beaten yolks. Add cool chicken broth, onion powder, and ground celery seed. Cook *over* (not in) hot water until mixture starts to thicken, stirring constantly. Remove from heat and add chopped hard-cooked eggs.

Low-Calory Soups

It is easy to be sensuous about soups. They smell good and there are so many garnishes to make them eye appealing. For a hearty lunch (with my homemade diet bread), or an appetizing first course for a party dinner, you can't beat soup!

WATERCRESS SOUP

2 bunches of watercress
2 cans chicken broth
2 chicken bouillon cubes
1 can evaporated skimmed milk
1 Tbsp flour

1 tsp onion powder
1 cup water
  (Grated lemon rind and
    paprika for garnish)

Put watercress, a little at a time, in blender with a little of the canned chicken broth. Add each until all the watercress is blended fine with all the chicken broth. Mix flour with water, a little at a time, until it's quite smooth and you have used all the water, then add the mixture slowly enough to the can of evaporated skimmed milk so that there are no lumps. Now put all the ingredients together and heat to just under boiling point, stirring all the while.

Let this mixture simmer about fifteen minutes, stirring it frequently. If the soup seems to need more salt, add another bouillon cube and mix until dissolved. If the soup seems a little thick, add a little skimmed milk. It is also very good served cold. This amount will serve six.

You can make a variety of delicious and unusual soups by substituting any of the following cooked vegetables for watercress: carrots, spinach, broccoli, cauliflower, asparagus.

For a fancy touch, garnish soup with any of these: finely chopped chives, cucumbers, pimientos, red or green sweet pepper, scallions; thinly sliced and peeled tomatoes or halved cherry tomatoes.

GREEK EGG LEMON SOUP

4 cups chicken broth
2 chicken bouillon cubes
3 eggs

Juice of one lemon
(Chopped parsley for garnish)

Use the top half of a double boiler right on the burner to heat the broth. Add the bouillon cubes and stir until dissolved. When the broth is hot, put hot water into the bottom part of double boiler and set the top half into it. Beat the eggs until very light and add the lemon juice to them.

Now take a cup of the broth and add it to the egg mixture, beating very slowly. Then add egg and broth mixture to the remainder of the broth in the top of the double boiler. Mix well. Place the lid on and let cook about ten minutes on *a very low flame.* (This mixture will curdle if placed directly over flame.) Serves four.

CREAMED MUSHROOM SOUP

1 pound of fresh mushrooms, cleaned

1 Tbsp onion powder

¼ tsp celery powder

2 cans chicken broth

3 chicken bouillon cubes

1 can evaporated skimmed milk

Water, if desired, for thinning

Place mushrooms in blender, a few at a time, with some of the chicken broth—blend until quite fine but not liquefied. Repeat until all the mushrooms have been used. Thin the evaporated milk, slowly, with the rest of the chicken broth. Then put all the ingredients together in a pot and heat slowly, stirring all the while, until soup comes to a boil. Turn down heat and let simmer five minutes, stirring occasionally. If this mixture seems too thick, add a little water, but taste it first, so that you don't thin it too much to weaken the flavor.

If you do add water, let it simmer a little longer. Garnish with lemon slices if you like. Serves six.

VEGETABLE SOUP

2 8-oz cans mixed vegetable juices (V8)

2 cans beef broth

2 beef bouillon cubes

2 Tbsp onion powder

2 cups cut-up celery

2 cups cut-up raw carrots

1 cup cut-up raw turnips

2 cups raw green string beans

½ cup chopped parsley

Put raw vegetables into blender with either beef broth or two cans of mixed vegetable juices (V8). Just blend enough to cut them up into small pieces. Then put all ingredients together and cook for fifteen minutes. Add a little water if too thick. Serves four.

ONION SOUP

2 medium peeled and thinly sliced onions

2 cans beef broth

3 beef bouillon cubes

4 very thin slices of French bread

4 Tbsp grated cheese

1 Tbsp butter

Brown onion powder in nonstick pan, stirring all the while, so it does not burn. Remove to pot for cooking soup. Melt butter in the same pan and brown slices of onion. Put all ingredients except bread and cheese together and simmer twenty minutes. Pour out four servings in ovenproof soup bowls. Place a slice of French bread on each, sprinkle with cheese, and place under broiler until light brown. Serve.

COLD BEET BORSCHT

1¼ cups water

4 beets

1 Tbsp sugar

Juice of one lemon

¼ cucumber chopped fine

1 tsp onion powder

¼ tsp celery powder

1 tsp chopped parsley

½ pint imitation sour cream (see Sauces, above), or

½ pint yogurt

Peel beets and put them a little at a time in blender with water. Don't let them get too fine. When you have blended all the beets with the water, add the sugar, onion, and celery powder in a pot and bring to a boil. Turn down heat and let simmer ten minutes. Remove from stove and when cool add lemon juice. Chill and before serving add some of the chopped cucumber to each bowl of borscht.

Add a dollop of yogurt (or sour cream) and sprinkle of parsley and serve. Serves four.

CREAM OF CELERY SOUP

6 stalks of celery
2 potatoes, peeled
1 tsp onion powder
½ tsp celery powder
7 or 8 sprigs parsley

1 Tbsp fresh dill, chopped,
   or 1 tsp dry dill weed
2 cups water
2 chicken bouillon cubes
1 can evaporated skim milk

Put potatoes and parsley in blender with enough water to liquefy. Now, dice the celery stalks rather fine. Mix remainder of water with the milk. Combine all the ingredients except the celery and simmer twenty minutes, adding the celery after the first ten minutes. Let simmer again until celery is tender. Serve with a teaspoon of chopped pimiento for garnish. Serves four.

TOMATO MADRILENE

2 cups tomato juice
2 cans chicken broth
2 chicken bouillon cubes

1 tsp onion powder
2 envelopes plain gelatin
¼ cup dry sherry

Soften gelatin in one-half cup of cold chicken broth. Combine remaining ingredients and let come to a boil. Turn heat down and let simmer. Remove from heat while you add softened gelatin to dissolve. Pour into a shallow pan and let chill until firm. To serve, cut into small cubes, pile into cups, and serve with a thin slice of lemon. Serves four.

For an elegant touch, top each bowl of madrilene with a tablespoon of my sour cream and a quarter teaspoon red caviar.

HOT BEET BORSCHT

2 cans beef broth
3 beef bouillon cubes
1 Tbsp onion powder

¼ tsp celery powder
6 beets
1 cup cabbage

Put beets and beef broth into blender and blend thoroughly, until beets are all used. Then add more broth and add the cabbage—again blending to fine. Transfer the mixture to a saucepan, add onion and celery powder and bouillon cubes, and bring to a boil. Reduce heat and let simmer about fifteen minutes. Serves six.

NEW ENGLAND CLAM CHOWDER

1 large can minced clams
1 Tbsp onion powder
¼ tsp celery powder
1 cup skimmed milk

1 can evaporated skimmed milk
2 chicken bouillon cubes
1 potato, peeled and chopped

Drain liquid from clams—put clams in pot for soup. Put clam juice in blender with chopped potato, blend until quite fine. Now mix skimmed milk with evaporated milk. Combine all ingredients in pot and let simmer for ten minutes, stirring fairly often. Sprinkle with chopped parsley and serve. Serves four.

MANHATTAN CLAM CHOWDER

1 large can minced clams
⅛ teaspoon sweet basil
⅛ tsp thyme
⅛ tsp bay leaf
1 Tbsp onion powder

¼ teaspoon celery powder
1 can chicken broth
1 chicken bouillon cube
1 No. 2 can tomatoes
1 large potato

Peel and dice potato. Cook them in chicken broth with bouillon cube added until potatoes are almost done. Add the remainder of the ingredients and let simmer for fifteen minutes. Serves six.

COLD CUCUMBER SOUP

2 cans chicken broth
2 chicken bouillon cubes
2 Tbsp onion powder
¼ tsp celery powder
3 cucumbers
¼ pint yogurt

Put cucumbers in blender with chicken broth. Let blend until fine but not liquefied; pour into saucepan, add celery and onion powder, then bouillon cubes. Bring to a boil, let simmer for five minutes. Remove from heat and chill. Serve with dollop of yogurt and sprinkle with chopped parsley and paprika. Serves six.

COLD FRUIT SOUP

1 cup canned sweet black
    cherries with juice
1 cup canned pitted sour
    cherries with juice
1 cup red wine
    Juice of ½ lemon
2 tsp cornstarch
1 cup water
    A few fresh strawberries,
    blueberries, or any fresh
    berries in season.

Moisten cornstarch with cold water and stir until all lumps are out. Add all the rest of the ingredients and all the remaining water. Bring to a boil. Reduce heat and let simmer ten minutes. Chill. Serve with a dollop of yogurt or my sour cream.

Entrees

BASIC MEAT LOAF

You can do much more with this basic receipe (p. 70) than just make a meat loaf. Here are some examples:

Meatballs: Roll the meat into balls about the size of a

golf ball. Brown them for five minutes in a little oil, then drain on paper towels and simmer them in your favorite tomato sauce for twenty minutes.

Swedish meatballs: Form into balls and brown, as above. Transfer the balls to a baking dish, top each with a tablespoon of yogurt or my sour cream, and bake for twenty-five minutes in a 350° oven.

Stuffed peppers: Cut the tops off as many green peppers as you require (two for each person). Remove seeds from peppers and stuff with the basic meat mixture. Arrange the peppers in a casserole dish. Replace the tops, and pour two cups of beef broth or tomato sauce over the peppers. Bake for thirty minutes in a 375° oven.

Barbecued Beef: Brown the meat mixture in a large frying pan (no oil is needed). Add two cups barbecue sauce and simmer for twenty minutes.

Stuffed Eggplant: Slice the eggplant in half, lengthwise. Slash the white meat several times with a knife and sprinkle with salt. Let stand fifteen minutes. Squeeze the juices from the eggplant and scoop out most of the meat with a spoon. Cut into small pieces and saute with the basic meat-loaf mixture until beef is thoroughly browned. Transfer meat and eggplant mixture back into eggplant shells. Arrange stuffed eggplant in a baking dish, meat-side up. Pour enough beef broth into the baking dish to cover one inch. Sprinkle with grated cheese and bake in a 350° oven for thirty minutes.

Joe's Special: A famous San Francisco dish. Thoroughly wash one pound of fresh spinach and tear the leaves into small pieces. Brown the meat thoroughly in a large skillet. Stir in the spinach and continue frying until the leaves are soft and wilted and have shrunk to about one-quarter their original size.

THE BASIC MEAT LOAF MIXTURE

1 pound lean ground beef
1 egg
1 Tbsp onion powder
1 tsp celery powder
1 tsp dry mustard
½ tsp salt
½ tsp pepper

½ cup yogurt
2 Tbsp hamburger relish
¼ cup catsup
½ tsp oregano
½ tsp thyme
1 tsp red pepper

Mix ingredients thoroughly, transfer to a baking dish, and put in a 400° oven for 40 minutes. If you are not using very lean beef, form the beef into a mound on top of a broiler pan. The fat will drip off as the meat cooks. Serves four.

SALMON LOAF

Sole, halibut, flounder, and just about any other fresh fish may be substituted for salmon in this recipe. Serve with Egg Sauce.

1 large can salmon, bones and
* skin removed*
1 Tbsp onion powder
1 tsp celery powder
½ cup plain yogurt

1 egg
¼ tsp salt
¼ tsp white pepper
Juice of 1 lemon

Mix the ingredients thoroughly, place in a greased loaf pan, and bake in a 375° oven for twenty-five minutes. *Variation:* Scoop the pulp and seeds out of four large, ripe tomatoes. Simmer the pulp in two cups of clam juice for five minutes. Stuff the salmon mixture into the tomatoes, transfer them to a baking dish, pour the clam juice mixture over it, and bake in a 375° oven for twenty-five minutes. Serves four.

Salmon loaf is delicious served cold on a bed of lettuce, with my mayonnaise.

CHICKEN LOAF

1½ cups chicken meat, cooked
    and ground in food
    grinder or blender
2 tsp onion powder
½ tsp celery powder

½ cup cooked mushrooms
¼ cup chicken broth
1 egg
Pinch saffron

Brown onion powder in an ungreased skillet. Combine all ingredients and mix thoroughly. Place in greased loaf pan and bake in 350° oven for thirty-five minutes. Serve with Lemon or Creole Sauce (see p. 61). Serves four.

VEAL MARSALA (WITH SAPSAGO)

1 pound veal scallops
⅓ cup grated Sapsago cheese
    (a cheese made from skim
    milk; substitute Parmesan
    cheese if you cannot
    obtain Sapsago)
1 cup fresh mushrooms,
    cleaned and diced

1 tsp onion powder
¼ tsp ground celery powder
¼ tsp oregano
1 chicken bouillon cube
⅓ cup Marsala wine
2 tsp cooking oil

Heat oil in nonstick skillet. Coat meat with grated cheese. Brown on both sides. Add remaining ingredients. Cover pan and simmer on low heat for 20 minutes. Serves two.

DEVILED EGG AND SHRIMP CASSEROLE

1 pound cooked cleaned
    shrimp
6 hard-boiled eggs
½ tsp Worcestershire sauce
2 tsp onion powder
½ tsp celery powder

1 chicken bouillon cube
¼ cup chicken broth
1 can evaporated skimmed
    milk
½ cup grated cheese
¼ cup sherry

Peel and halve eggs. Dissolve chicken bouillon cube in chicken broth. Add one teaspoon onion powder, ¼ teaspoon celery powder, and the Worcestershire sauce. Mash egg yolks and moisten thoroughly with bouillon mix. Fill whites with the mixture. Place eggs in bottom of casserole. Mix evaporated milk with one teaspoon onion powder and the other ¼ teaspoon celery powder. Gradually mix in sherry. Cover eggs with shrimp. Pour milk mixture over whole, then sprinkle with cheese and place under broiler until lightly browned. Serves four.

CRAB OR LOBSTER ORIENTAL

1 pound cooked lobster or
    crab meat
½ cup water chestnuts,
    sliced thin
½ cup bamboo shoots
1 tsp onion powder
¼ tsp celery powder

1 Tbsp cornstarch
½ cup canned button
    mushrooms
1 Tbsp chopped chives
2 cups chicken broth
2 chicken bouillon cubes
1½ Tbsp soy sauce

Dissolve chicken bouillon cubes in chicken broth. Add soy sauce, celery powder, and onion powder. Add a few tablespoons of this liquid slowly to the cornstarch, mixing very smooth. Add the cornstarch mixture to the broth. Stir constantly, over heat, until mixture thickens. Add lobster or crab meat. Let simmer five minutes. Then add mushrooms, water chestnuts, and bamboo shoots. Simmer two minutes longer.

STUFFED LOBSTER TAILS

4 cooked lobster tails
1 tsp onion powder
¼ tsp celery powder

⅓ cup dry sherry
½ can evaporated skimmed
    milk

Remove lobster meat from shell; save the shells. Mix onion powder, celery powder and sherry together. Add skimmed evaporated milk. Heat over low flame. Add lobster chunks.

Mix so, that all lobster chunks are covered. Restuff the shells and place under broiler until just light brown. Serves two.

CHICKEN HELEN

3 cups cooked chicken meat	2 chicken bouillon cubes
1 tsp onion powder	1 can evaporated skimmed milk
½ tsp celery powder	
Pinch of saffron	2 tsp flour

Dissolve chicken cubes in ½ cup milk; mix in the flour slowly, to avoid lumps. When smooth, add remainder of milk plus other ingredients, except for the chicken. Put in two-quart sauce pan over heat, stirring continuously until mixture thickens. Add chicken. Cook another five minutes. Serves four.

FEGATO VENEZIANA

This is a good way to get your family to eat liver without realizing it. Kidneys, sweetbreads, brains, heart, and other low-calory, high-nutrient foods that are often disliked may be disguised in the same way.

1 pound calves' liver, cut into 1-inch cubes	2 cups tomato sauce
	1 tsp salt
1 onion, sliced	1 tsp celery powder
1 clove garlic, minced	1 tsp hot sauce
2 green peppers, chopped	1 tsp dry mustard
2 tomatoes, chopped	1 tsp tarragon

Sauté the onions, garlic and green pepper in two tablespoons oil until the onions are a pale yellow and the peppers are tender. Remove from pan and drain well on paper towels. In a clean, ungreased skillet, heat the tomato sauce. Add the tomatoes, peppers, onions, and mushrooms and bring to a simmer. Add seasonings and liver. Simmer, covered, for fifteen minutes. Serves four.

KIDNEYS KINGSTON ROAD

Another way of disguising an unpopular food. Substitute liver for kidneys if desired.

8 lamb or veal kidneys	2 tsp onion powder
2 Tbsp butter	½ tsp celery powder
1 cup yogurt	1 tsp tarragon
1 Tbsp prepared mustard	½ cup chicken broth
1 tsp dry mustard	½ cup chopped parsley
1 Tbsp tarragon vinegar	

Remove the filament from the kidneys (or have your butcher do it). Brown the kidneys on both sides in the butter. They will not become truly brown, like beef, but will turn a light gray and be spongy to the touch. This will only take a few minutes on each side.

Drain the kidneys thoroughly on paper towels. Slice them diagonally into ¼-inch slices. To preserve the precious juices, slice them on a plate or in a wooden chopping bowl.

Brown the onion and celery powder in an ungreased non-stick skillet. Add the remaining ingredients plus the kidneys, and simmer, covered, for twenty minutes. Serves two.

LOW-CALORY CURRY

Chicken, beef, lamb, shrimp, lobster—all can be curried with ease. Don't overlook currying liver and kidneys, too: another tricky way of slipping slimming, nutrient-packed meat into your menu.

¼ cup curry powder	1 cup broth (beef, chicken, or clam juice, depending upon which meat you use).
2 tsp onion powder	
1 tsp celery powder	
1 tsp coriander	½ cup tomato paste
1 tsp turmeric	1 cup grated, unsweetened coconut
1 tsp Cayenne pepper	
1 tsp dried mustard	2 lbs cooked meat (your choice)
1 cup plain yogurt	

Brown the curry, onion, and celery powder in an ungreased nonstick pan. Add the remaining ingredients *except the meat and coconut* and bring to a simmer. Let the mixture simmer for 30 minutes, adding more broth if necessary.

Add the meat and simmer until the meat is tender, again adding more broth if necessary. If the meat is precooked it only needs to warm through. Raw shrimp and liver will be done in ten minutes. Raw beef, lamb, veal, and chicken will require 30 to 60 minutes of additional simmering.

Spoon mixture onto plates and sprinkle with grated coconut. Serves four. Chutney is the traditional garnish for a curry, but it's expensive and high in calories. Here is a substitute:

LOW-CALORY CHUTNEY

1 cup canned apricots, drained	½ cup brown sugar
1 cup canned peaches, drained	1 cup beef broth
1 cup canned tomatoes, with juice	1 cup raisins, soaked in warm water and drained
1 cup chopped onion	1 tsp dry mustard
1 cup finely chopped green pepper	2 Tbsp curry powder
	½ cup red vinegar

Chop apricots, peaches, and tomatoes coarsely. Mix all the ingredients except the beef broth and place them in a saucepan and bring them to a gentle boil. Simmer for 20 minutes, adding beef broth if necessary to prevent drying. Serve cold or hot.

Serve the curry and chutney with a variety of side relishes: chopped cucumber, mustard pickles, raisins, slivered almonds, and the many varieties of *sombols* you'll find at your gourmet shop.

MANDARIN PORK CHOPS

Yes, you can have pork chops. For years, even the most sensible authors of diet books have arbitrarily eliminated pork from the dieter's menu: I don't know why. If trimmed of fat and cooked properly, a lean pork chop has fewer calories than chicken, beef, lamb, or veal (according to some charts) and is much higher in vitamin B than these other meats. But remember: Broil it and trim off all visible fat.

Here is an elegant recipe for pork chops:

1 pound fresh, cooked spinach	8 lean pork chops
2 cups mandarin oranges, drained	1 Tbsp dried mint
1 Tbsp horseradish	1 cup beef broth

Mix the horseradish, mandarin orange slices, and beef broth together in a saucepan. Bring to a gentle boil and keep warm until serving time.

Rub the pork chops with the dried mint and broil 10 to 15 minutes on each side, depending on thickness of chops.

Cook the spinach and place it on a serving bowl or individual plates. Arrange the pork chops on top of the spinach and spoon the mandarin orange mixture over them. Serves four.

BAKED EGGS FLORENTINE

1½ pounds fresh spinach	½ cup chicken broth
1 cup evaporated skim milk	4 eggs (number varies with number of people being served).
½ cup cooked mushroom pieces	

Cook the spinach in the customary manner. If frozen spinach is used, be sure to remove stems before cooking. You will need two to three packages of frozen spinach.

Mix the cooked spinach with the milk, mushrooms, and broth. Use less milk if the mixture begins to look a bit soupy.

Put the spinach mixture into a casserole dish. With a glass or soup ladle, make depressions about the size of an egg.

Crack the eggs one by one onto a saucer and carefully pour them into the holes you prepared in the spinach mixture.

Sprinkle with paprika or grated cheese and bake, uncovered, in a 350° oven for 20 minutes (shorter for softer yolks, longer for harder yolks). Serves four.

MINTY LAMB CHOPS

4 loin lamb chops   *1 Tbsp rosemary*
1 Tbsp dry mint   *Apricot dressing (see below)*

Carefully trim all visible fat from the lamb chops. Rub the mint and rosemary into the meat and place in refrigerator for one hour, occasionally turning the meat and rubbing the herbs in again.

Broil the lamb chops to desired degree of doneness (ten minutes on each side for medium-rare chops of moderate thickness). Serve with Apricot Dressing and unpeeled zucchini, thinly sliced and simmered in beef broth for seven minutes. Serves two.

APRICOT DRESSING

1 can apricots, drained *1 tsp dry mustard*
1 cup beef broth   *¼ cup finely chopped*
1 tsp dry mint   *scallions*

Bring the mixture to a gentle boil and simmer for seven minutes.

LOW-CALORY BEEF STEW

Lamb or chicken may be substituted for beef in this make-in-minutes recipe.

2 carrots, thinly sliced
1 jar small white onions, drained
3 stalks celery, chopped
1 large onion, coarsely chopped
2 green peppers, coarsely chopped
2 tomatoes, coarsely chopped
1 box frozen peas

2 pounds flank steak, cut in 1½-inch squares
2 cups beef broth
1 Tbsp cooking oil
1 tsp salt
½ tsp pepper
1 tsp dry mustard
½ tsp tarragon
1 Tbsp flour

Dust the meat with flour and brown quickly on all sides in the cooking oil. Drain the meat on paper towels. Place meat and beef broth in deep skillet or heavy saucepan and simmer for thirty minutes. Add vegetables and herbs and simmer an additional thirty minutes. Thicken with arrowroot or cornstarch if desired. Serves six.

LOW-CALORY DESSERTS

If you tried yogurt once and didn't like it, I urge you to try it again. I myself didn't like the old-fashioned kind that had raspberries, strawberries, or whatever in a syrupy mess at the bottom of the container. Today you can find delicious yogurts made from skim milk and delicately flavored with lemon, orange, cinnamon apple, pineapple, strawberries, blueberries, etc. These are premixed and have a wonderful texture. Serve them in champagne glasses topped with a little fresh fruit. Use your imagination to dream up all sorts of exotic combinations. For example, the cinnamon apple yogurt mixed with horseradish is great with pork chops.

MERINGUE SHELL

4 egg whites

¼ cup granulated sugar

⅛ tsp cream of tartar

1 tsp vanilla

1 tsp vinegar

Add vinegar to egg whites and beat until frothy. Add the cream of tartar and beat until the egg whites form soft peaks. Add the vanilla and then the sugar, a tablespoon at a time. Continue beating until the whites become very stiff.

Scoop the meringue onto a pie tin lined with brown paper. Form a shell with the aid of a rubber spatula. Bake in a 325° oven for one hour. Turn off the oven. *Do not open it.* Let the meringue remain in the oven until it is room temperature. Then fill it with any of the following recipes.

CHOCOLATE SPONGE

4 oz German sweet chocolate

⅓ cup evaporated skimmed
     milk

2 tsp vanilla

1 tsp unflavored gelatin

¼ cup cold water

4 eggs

Place gelatin in cold water, then dissolve the mixture in heated evaporated milk. Put this mixture in the top of a double boiler with the chocolate. Heat, stirring constantly, until the chocolate has melted.

Separate the eggs. Beat yolks until very thick and light. Add the beaten yolks and vanilla and heat over the double boiler for 2 minutes. Remove from heat.

Beat the egg whites until stiff and fold into the chocolate mixture. Cool in refrigerator, stirring with the spatula every 15 minutes. When the mixture is about to "set" (in about 45 minutes), spoon it into the meringue shell. Return to refrigerator for at least 2 hours.

79

STRAWBERRY CHIFFON

1 can evaporated skimmed
    milk
1 Tbsp unflavored gelatin

¼ cup cold water
1 package frozen strawberries

Soak gelatin in cold water, Add milk and heat in the top of a double boiler until gelatin is completely dissolved. Remove from heat.

When cool, place in the refrigerator until the mixture starts to thicken. Chop the partially frozen berries and add them to the mixture; beat until mixture forms soft peaks and nearly doubles in size. Spoon into the meringue shell and refrigerate for at least two hours. Any frozen fruits may be substituted for strawberries.

MAPLE CREAM CHIFFON

1 can evaporated skimmed
    milk
1 Tbsp unflavored gelatin

¼ cup cold water
½ cup maple syrup
1 tsp maple or rum flavoring

Follow the instructions for Strawberry Chiffon (*above*) but at the last step add maple syrup and flavoring instead of strawberries.

NOTE: These recipes may be used as puddings, without the meringue shell. If you freeze them they make a delicious low-calorie substitute for ice cream.

How to Resist the Restaurant Ruse

The most belabored dodge for avoiding caution in the selection of low-calory dinners is the old restaurant ruse of contending that if you have to eat out you've got to stay fat.

That wasn't true ten years ago and it's certainly not true now. And you don't have to go to "health" restaurants to eat nutritious, low-calory food, either. With a few basic facts about menu reading you can go to the humblest or the most elaborate restaurant without fear.

The infamous lunch hour

The office worker—be he stock-room clerk or chief executive, typist or fashion model—faces the problem of the lunch hour five days a week. It should be a pleasure, not a problem. It can be if you follow these suggestions.

Are you eating a good breakfast? If you are, you will feel more alert during the morning hours, and when lunch time comes you will not be ravenously hungry.

Can you take your lunch with you? If you can, by all means do. You needn't do this every day of the week. If you start taking your lunch with you, if you get into the habit of preparing it the night before and keeping it in the refrigerator, you will be more than half way to winning the battle with the restaurant ruse. Eat your lunch at your desk, or, if it's a nice day, go to a nearby park. When you've finished you will have time to shop, visit a museum or exhibition, read a magazine—or just take a healthful, refreshing walk.

You can make sandwiches with thinly sliced bread and some of the spreads in the chapter "Dips and Snacks." You can prepare a vitamin-packed tossed green salad or a fruit salad and pack them in plastic cartons—the kind cole slaw and potato salad come in. You can bring cold cuts, vegetables, fruits. You can make delicious tuna, shrimp, crab, lobster, salmon, chicken, and ham salads with my low-calorie mayonnaise, some chopped celery, green pepper, and pimiento, and a little onion powder. You can bring bouillon cubes and make your own broth (and coffee and tea). You can carry cold drinks and hot soups in a thermos bottle.

When you bring your own lunch you spare yourself the time lost at a crowded restaurant; you save money; and you know exactly what you're getting!

When you lunch out

It may not be practical for you to take your lunch to work. There are situations that require you to eat out.

If you're the typical worker and not on an expense account you will usually be eating in typical luncheonette. Avoid pizza parlors; a few slices of pizza and a soda may be cheap but it's not going to do you a bit of good.

Today so many chic people demand low-calorie foods that most restaurants—particularly luncheonettes—are forced to carry them.

Look at the menu. You'll probably find a "Dieters Special." If not, you'll surely find various salad platters. When ordering, say, a shrimp salad platter, ask that the potato salad be omitted. Announce in a clear voice that you do not want bread—and if the waitress brings it anyway, make her take it back. Out of sight, out of mind.

There is always the inevitable hamburger, which you will order without bread, and with a tomato and lettuce salad, without dressing. You don't know what's in the hamburger— it may be made from the fattest cut of meat—but that's the risk you take when you eat out.

Bring your own salad dressing with you. Choose one of my recipes that appeals to you, and pour a few tablespoons into an empty herb or spice bottle. Keep it in your purse or pocket, and when the salad comes, dress it yourself. Remember, you don't know how long the luncheonette's salad dressing has been sitting around, who made it, or how many people have had their fingers in it. All you do know is that it's full of fat.

For dessert ask for a fruit cup. If they don't have one, pick up an apple or a pear or a banana or a peach or a cup of flavored yogurt on your way back to the office. If you're forbidden to eat it at your desk, take it to the powder room.

The expense-account trap

Executives and others on expense accounts have the unfortunate problem of an excess of luxury. They may not want to eat any lunch at all . . . and then find they have to take a visiting fireman to a high-class restaurant for a business lunch. The martinis flow and the calory intake jumps.

The first thing such people should do is forget about preluncheon cocktails forever. There's no rule that says you have *got* to have a drink before lunch. If the person you're taking wants one, buy him one. That's good business.

But don't feel any obligation to join him. One cocktail usually leads to two—and the afternoon is shot. That's not good business.

If the others are drinking you can order fresh fruit juice (or tomato or clam) or a low-calorie soda, iced tea, iced coffee, or just plain soda with lemon. (With the calories you saved during the cocktail hour you can treat yourself to one of those delicious pumpernickel rolls.)

Dining out can be a treat

What about dinner? What about the special occasion when you want to splurge, when you want to treat yourself to a really sumptuous meal at a famous restaurant? Can you do it the natural way?

Certainly. Again, just observe a few simple rules and you can dine in style.

The worst high-calorie crimes committed in restaurants are those committed during the first fifteen or twenty minutes after arrival—from waiting for a drink through the first course.

When you go into the restaurant you are hungry, and all of your senses are being stimulated by the sight and sound and smells of the food being served around you.

First the waiter usually brings rolls and butter to your table and takes your cocktail order.

Now is the time to declare for the thin man. Before you order your drink, decide if you are going to have an appetizer and/or a salad. If you are, ask the waiter to bring it or them to your table immediately, even before your cocktail. Get some nonstarch food into you from the start. Ask that the bread be taken away. If there are others, eat steadily at your salad or shrimp cocktail or oysters and ignore the bread.

Be firm, don't mumble, speak up so that your waiter knows that you know what you want. In most restaurants, appetizers, soup, and salad don't take as long as the drink. So again, make sure that your waiter knows that at least one of these dishes is to be served before, or at least with, the cocktail.

This device alone will save you hundreds of calories each week.

The cocktail crisis

The kind of cocktail you order is important. The effect of alcohol on the body is described in detail in the chapter "Lose With Booze." Here I'll just say this; on a special occasion it is pleasant to have a cocktail before dinner. It relaxes you and stimulates your appetite. But try to limit yourself to one—you came to the restaurant to sample the food, remember? Not to get drunk. Prefer a highball, but if you must have a martini, say, or a Manhattan, order it "on the rocks," and when your waiter asks if you want another, say no, thanks, just a little more ice, please.

Reading the menu

Reading menus can be a source of great pleasure in and of itself. Keep an eye out for the low-calory foods and you'll have even more fun beating the menu makers at their own game.

In a good American restaurant you can always find superb low-calory appetizers such as:

Melon	Clam Juice
Cherrystone clams	Grapefruit
Marinated herring	Shrimp cocktail
(without sour cream)	Crab meat cocktail
Tomato juice	

You will find such low-calory soups as:

Bouillon, hot or cold	Jellied madrilene
Beet borscht (no sour cream)	Tomato bouillon
Garden vegetable soup	Onion soup

Order your tossed green salad without dressing. If it embarrasses you to pour your own dressing from your own bottle, ask the waiter to mix a special dressing for you of one teaspoon oil, one teaspoon lemon juice, and one teaspoon water. Commander Whitehead, the famed tycoon, always does this, and the dressing has come to be known as "Whitehead Dressing" in many of the restaurants he patronizes.

Another salad tip; ask for watercress salad instead of ordinary salad. Your waiter will be impressed at your worldly wisdom.

The main course is easy; the average menu of a good American restaurant will list a variety of fish and meat. You cannot do better to have them baked or broiled to enjoy the full flavor of their natural goodness.

If potatoes are served, ask if you can substitute another vegetable (zucchini, green beans, broccoli, etc.). A small pat of butter on this vegetable won't kill you . . . but why not try a few drops of lemon juice or your own low-calory dressing instead?

If you are not permitted to substitute a low-calory vegetable, ask that the potatoes be omitted from your plate, and insist on a salad whether it is included in your meal or not. Hang the expense.

When it comes time for dessert, stick to a fresh fruit cup. It may not be on the menu, but if the restaurant is worth its salt it will be able to whip one up for you.

Alternatives for dessert: custard, iced coffee (sweetened with saccharin), mousse, or sherbet.

10   Lose With Booze

Just as we were told for years that we could not eat pork and stay slim, so we were told for years that we could not drink and stay slim.

Then along came an article in *Esquire* magazine that pointed out that alcohol had no fat—and *then* came a series of books telling us how to drink and stay slim. And so we started drinking and we started getting fat.

What is the truth? Here it is:

- Alcohol *does not* contain fat.
- Alchol *does* contain calories.
- Alcohol—that is, most drinks—does contain sugar which is converted to fat in your body.
- Alcohol has *no food value*.
- Alcohol used in place of food will cause serious damage to your health.
- Alcohol relaxes you, lowers your ability to resist food, and often stimulates the appetite.
- You *can* drink—*in moderation*—and stay healthy and slim.

What is moderation?

We drink to relax. We drink to be convivial. We drink to celebrate. We drink because there are situations (*we think!*)

in which it would be embarrassing not to drink. We drink to forget our problems. We—or some of us—use drinking as a shortcut to being ourselves.

In short, we drink for as many different reasons as we are ourselves different—perhaps for the same reasons that we eat more than we should.

How many calories in a martini?

Whatever your reasons for drinking, you can indeed continue to drink, *in moderation,* and stay slim. But don't kid yourself: When you take a drink, you're taking calories.

It is true that most drinks are lower in calories than cakes, pies, and other rich desserts. But drinks are far higher in calories than half a grapefruit or a slice of melon.

Trading calories

If you want to drink and stay slim, you must learn to trade the calories in food for the calories in alcohol. This kind of trading can be most pleasant, but you must be careful not to trade your protein- and mineral-filled calories for those in liquor. This leads to trouble—liver damage, kidney damage, nervousness, and general malnutrition.

When you take a drink ask yourself two things:

(1) How many calories are there in this drink and how can I reduce them?

(2) What high-calory, low-nutrient food can I give up in favor of my drink?

The dangerous three

Liqueurs, beer, and wine are the dangerous three. They have sugar in them as well as alcohol and are higher in calories than straight distilled spirits.

Take beer. It is lower in its percentage of alcohol than wine or distilled spirits, and it contains 14 calories an ounce, compared to 90-proof gin, which has 90 calories per ounce. Few people would consider an ounce of beer a serious drink. Yet a 12-ounce can of beer contains about 170 calories—nearly twice that of a gin-and-low-calory-tonic highball (95 calories).

If *wines* play an important part in your life, remember that a four-ounce glass of most wines contains as many calories as an eight-ounce glass of lager beer (and sometimes more). Even four ounces of a dry white wine such as Liebfraumilch, which is only 10-percent alcohol, has 84 calories—more than an ounce of 80-proof vodka on the rocks.

Keep this in mind: Red wines are generally higher in calories than white wines, and sweet wines are always higher in calories than dry wines.

Light ale has fewer calories than heavy ale. Lager beer has fewer calories than bock beer. Ale generally has fewer calories than beer.

Try to forget about *liqueurs* altogether. These are usually taken after a meal, but since you are drinking to relax, the alcohol in them will do little to help you feel rosy since the food in your stomach will absorb much of it. When your host offers you a liqueur, ask if you may have a scotch and soda instead. This is just as acceptable as a liqueur and your host should have no objections, since it's less expensive. Better yet, ask for another cup of coffee. At home a glass of skim milk or fruit juice makes a fine nightcap.

Calories and cocktails

Your best bet for a quick pick-me-up after a long day's work is a highball or a cocktail. Here you have hundreds of choices; creative bartenders across the world have dreamed up all kinds of exotic concoctions to tempt you. Here are some guidelines to help resist them:

(1) Prefer 80-proof liquor to 86-, 90-, or 100-proof. It's cheaper and lower in calories.

(2) Remember this rule when drinking whiskey, vodka, gin, and most other distilled spirits: Each ounce of liquor contains one calory for every degree of proof. If you're drinking 80-proof vodka, you're getting 80 calories per ounce; if you're drinking 100-proof vodka, you're getting 100 calories per ounce.

(3) Prefer dry manhattans to sweet manhattans; prefer dry martinis to regular martinis, and vodka martinis to gin martinis.

(4) Always order cocktails "on the rocks." They'll stay cold longer, and as the ice melts the alcohol will be diluted—you'll get just as relaxed, but you'll spend more time on the drink, and will be less tempted to have a second (or third).

(5) Prefer highballs to cocktails. The mixes—wine, sugar, juice, cream, whatever—add more calories than ever . . . and besides, a highball takes longer to drink.

(6) Highballs should be mixed with water, soda, or a low-calory soft drink. (You can make your own low-calory tonic water by adding 2 teaspoons lemon juice to 6 ounces of club soda.)

(7) Avoid the exotic but extraneous garnishes many bartenders (including home bartenders) add to cocktails: maraschino cherries, olives, etc. Waitresses often place an order with a bartender this way: "One old-fashioned without the garbage." These ornaments *are* garbage as far as your stomach is concerned. If you must have something decorative with your drink, use a lemon peel or a cocktail onion.

(8) When "trading" calories, ask yourself this: "Am I getting the best deal in this trade?" If you're giving up the calories in a steak or salad for the calories in a martini, you're cheating yourself and endangering your health. If you're trading the calories in a roll, a potato, or a rich dessert, you're all right—providing you eat that steak and salad.

Don't delay dinner

(9) When ordering your drink (or making it at home) be sure that dinner is under way. Too many careless drinkers blame lazy waiters or forgetful wives or thoughtless hostesses for that second, or third, or fourth drink. If you're dining at a friend's house, there's not much you can do about hurrying up the dinner *except:* (a) Ask for more ice or more water and drink more slowly; and (b) If your friend has the habit of a prolonged cocktail hour, plan to arrive late—*very* late, if necessary.You're being no more rude than your host. There is nothing polite about forcing guests to sit through two or three hours of drinking before serving them dinner.

(10) It is both pleasant and wise to have snacks while you are enjoying the cocktail hour. They keep you from attacking the dinner like a starving refugee, and they counter the hazardous effects of alcohol on an empty or nearly empty stomach. But often too many of these snacks—pretzels, potato chips, crackers, creamy dips—are your enemies, high in calories, low in nutrients. There's not much you can do about this when you're at the home of a friend. But when entertaining yourself you can serve a good many tasty and applause-winning canapes and appetizers that will keep the hunger pangs down without keeping your weight up. Here are some suggestions and recipes for these snacks and dips.

Appetizers

The cocktail hour can break an otherwise low-calory day, so keep a good supply of nutritious, low-calory snacks on hand to keep your calory intake down.

It's not a good idea to drink on an empty stomach. You get intoxicated quickly, your resistance lowers, and you either develop an uncontrollable appetite or lose interest in food altogether. Either way, it's at the expense of your health.

Here are some novel recipes for dips and canapes—and some unusual items to dip into the dips in place of crackers, potato chips, pretzels, and the like.

Low-calory snacks to dunk in dips

Use fresh, crisp, cool vegetables, attractively cut and arranged on a platter around the dipping bowl.

Broccoli flowerettes

Carrot sticks

Cauliflowerettes

Celery sticks

Cherry tomatoes

Cucumber sticks or slices

Plum tomatoes

Belgian endive leaves

Fennel sticks

Turnip sticks

Cold meat strips

Thin slices of salami (rolled)

Thin slices of prosciutto ham (rolled)

Chilled shrimp

Crab legs

Lobster chunks

Tiny meat balls

Fresh pineapple chunks

Radishes

Low-calory dips

You can either spread these dips into celery sticks or radish roses, or put them in a bowl surrounded by a variety of the vegetables or meats.

Use my basic low-calory sour cream (p. 58) for all of these dips.

PIMENTO AND CHILI DIP

½ cup my sour cream
¼ cup chili sauce
1 tsp onion powder
¼ tsp celery powder

1 tsp dill weed
1 Tbsp drained chopped
    pimiento

Mix all ingredients and chill.

SEAFOOD DIP

¼ lb crab meat
¼ lb shrimp, cooked and cut
    up
1 cup my sour cream

1 tsp onion powder
¼ tsp ground celery seed
1 dash hot sauce
¼ cup chili sauce

Mix all ingredients and chill.

TUNA DIP

1 6-oz can tuna (water-
    packed), minced
2 Tbsp sweet pickle relish
1 tsp onion powder

½ tsp celery powder
¾ cup my sour cream
2 hard-cooked eggs (minced)
½ tsp salt

Combine all ingredients and chill.

MINCED CLAM DIP

1 can minced clams, drained
1 cup my sour cream
1 tsp lemon juice

1 tsp onion powder
½ tsp celery powder
¼ cup chili sauce

Combine all ingredients and chill.

TONGUE AND HORSERADISH DIP

¼ lb cooked smoked tongue
½ cup my sour cream

1 tsp onion powder
Salt to taste

Put all ingredients into a blender. Blend well and chill.

CRAB AND BACON DIP

1 lb lump crabmeat	½ cup chili sauce
1 package onion-and-bacon powdered dip mix	½ tsp tarragon vinegar
	½ tsp celery powder
½ tsp dry mustard	1½ cups my sour cream.

Thoroughly mix all ingredients except the crab meat. Then blend in the crab meat carefully, leaving attractive lumps in the dip.

CHICKEN DIP

2 cups cooked, white chicken meat	½ cup my sour cream
	1 hard-cooked egg
¼ tsp celery powder	¼ cup chopped green pepper
½ tsp onion powder	¼ cup chopped pimiento

Put all ingredients except chicken into the blender. Blend until very smooth. Add chicken and blend just a little longer—to mince the meat but not liquefy it. Chill and serve.

Low-calory canapes

Here are several tasty appetizers to serve when you grow weary of dips.

- Shrimp, crabmeat, or lobster meat nestled on a cooked artichoke leaf and topped with my mayonnaise or lemon juice.
- Braunschweiger on Melba toast.
- Smoked salmon on cucumber slices.
- Deviled eggs (made with my mayonnaise)
- Minimeatballs (see p. 68) in a chafing dish
- All-beef frankfurters cut in 1-inch slices and served with hot mustard.

94

- Sardines (boneless and skinless, packed in water) served on thinly sliced, raw zucchini.
- Stuffed mushrooms (stuff caps with my basic meat loaf mixture and broil for 5 to 7 minutes).

How to find more low-calory recipes

The recipes in this book will give you a good start on creating a host of recipes of your own. You've now learned the basic techniques of low-calory cooking, and you should be able to apply them to many of your favorite recipes.

But there are many, many other sources of low-calory recipes available to you today. Go to your book store or library and ask to be shown a few of the dozens of cookbooks now in print that are devoted exclusively to slimming foods.

The next time you're at the supermarket, browse through the magazine section. You'll find any number of women's magazines that carry a special section on low-calory dishes—and one magazine (*Weight Watchers*) that contains nothing but low-calory recipes.

11 Nature's Calory Counter

WE'RE SO LUCKY TODAY—those of us who want to stay slim and healthy. Not only do we know more about the thin foods; not only is it stylish to be thin; our whole attitude toward eating has changed.

When I was a child, back in the dark ages of the groaning board, a Thanksgiving or Christmas feast nearly killed all who participated in it. It was considered obligatory to use three or four dozen eggs, several pounds of butter, nuts, chocolate, three quarts of whipping cream, sausage, chicken and turkey livers and giblets in the preparation of the turkey dressing, vegetables, desserts (desserts *plural* mind you, not just one).

The guests would arrive and all would be gay and talk and laugh until they had ploughed through that Gargantuan meal. Then they would sit like graven images, unable to speak, desperately trying to hold their eyes open until they passed into a coma to sleep it off. No alcoholic ever had a worse hangover than those poor, tortured stuffers.

Fortunately, those deadly feasts are, for the most part, a thing of the past. More and more people are realizing that convivial gatherings and elegant entertaining don't mean serving heavy, stuffing, and stultifying foods.

Most people now realize that the presentation of such a meal to guests is not a favor, but a shove toward the grave.

Today all *sensible* hostesses are exerting a greater effort to select a menu for guests that is really more delicious. The lightness of the dinner lets us do the thing that we gather for —rekindle friendship through communication.

As we eat less it is more important than ever to make sure we get the necessary vitamins and minerals necessary to keep at the peak of health.

In this book you will find a number of recipes that are low in calories but high in nutrients. Yet I know that you have many favorite foods and recipes of your own. How many calories are in them? How many nutrients?

The **Color Calory Counter** I have prepared for you will help you determine just what foods you should choose and what foods you should avoid. The foods that are *lowest in calories and highest in nutrients* are printed in red. When you feel a craving for a fatty food, look through this chart. See if you can't find something equally appetizing and satisfying from the red entries. Practice the art of substitution as often as you can and you will be well on the way to a healthier, more attractive you.

When you substitute, keep these things in mind:

- Don't limit yourself to one kind of food. Select a variety —remember that the protein found in vegetables is not a complete protein; you need meat too, and you need a variety of vitamins and minerals.

- Don't regard this chart as the final word on vitamin and mineral content. Where the foods were grown or produced, how fresh they are, how they are prepared all determine the final amount of vitamins and minerals that ultimately enter your system.

- If you must eat a rich food, choose a rich food that is high in nutrients.

- In selecting your foods, try to get the daily minimum requirement of vitamins suggested by the Department of Agriculture.

Don't starve yourself. If you want to go on a 10-day wonder diet, consult your doctor. If you want a sensible, safe, permanent weight-loss program, see to it that you get 2700 calories a day. Stick to my menus, stick to the red-letter foods, and you won't have to worry about counting calories or vitamins at all. It's the natural way.

FOR YOUR CONVENIENCE in using the following charts, foods that are low in calories but high in vitamins and minerals *are printed in red.*

Bear in mind that the quoted percentages in all such charts may at times seem contradictory. These figures are necessarily drawn from a variety of sources in order to give you as complete a list as possible. Moreover, the amount of vitamins or minerals found in a given food may vary slightly from carrot to carrot — or even from laboratory to laboratory.

Do not use these charts as a rigid guide. The apple you eat may have more or less vitamins or calories than the one used by science. Rather use the chart as a general guide to the kinds of foods to avoid and the kinds of foods to favor. Use it as a general indication, one that is perfectly accurate within reasonable margins, of your caloric intake.

SOURCES: Chatfield, C. and Adams, G., *Approximate Composition of American Food Materials,* Handbook No. 8, U.S. Department of Agriculture, 1964; Booher, L. E., Hartzler, E. R., and Hewston, E. M., *Compilation of Vitamin Values,* U.S. Department of Agriculture Bulletin 638; and *Report of the Food and Nutrition Board,* National Academy of Sciences, National Research Council (revised edition, 1964); also miscellaneous publications of the Committee on Foods and Nutrition of the National Research Council.

Legend:
I.U.: *international units;* Mg: *milligrams;* Gr: *grams;* Tr: *trace;* O: *no contents.* Dash (–) means *information not available,* (not *no contents*).

Vitamins

Food Product	Portions	Calories	A (I.U.)	Thiamin	B Group (Mg) Ribo-Flavin	Niacin
Fruit						
Apples, raw	½ cup	60	45	.03	.02	.10
Applesauce, w/sugar	½ cup	88	40	.03	.04	Tr
unsweetened	½ cup	47	40	.03	.03	Tr
*Apricots, raw	½ cup	51	2700	.03	.04	.6
w/syrup	½ cup	95	2600	.02	.03	.4
Banana, raw	6½ inches	73	160	.04	.05	.6
Blackberries						
unsweetened	½ cup	86	210	.02	.02	.2
frozen, sweetened	½ cup	110	160	.02	.11	.7
Blueberries, raw	½ cup	71	115	.03	.07	.6
w/syrup	½ cup	113	40	.02	.02	.2
frozen, sweetened	½ cup	120	35	.05	.06	.5
*Cantaloup, medium	¼ melon	81	9230	.11	.08	1.6
Cassaba melon	⅛ melon	54	60	.08	.06	1.2
Cherries, raw, sweet	½ cup	80	130	.06	.07	.5
Cherries, w/syrup	½ cup	114	40	.02	0	0
Cherries, frozen, sweetened	½ cup	126	550	.03	.07	.3
Crabapples, raw	¼ cup	39	25	.02	.01	tr
Cranberries, raw	½ cup	53	45	.03	.02	tr
sauce	¼ cup	115	20	.02	.02	.1
Currants red & white raw	1 cup	114	275	.09	.11	.2
Dates	2 large or 3 small	156	30	.05	.06	1.3
Figs, raw	1 small	46	45	.03	.03	.2
Figs, dried	½ cup	312	90	.12	.12	.8
Figs w/syrup	3 figs	136	60	.03	.04	.4
Fruit cocktail in syrup	½ cup	81	180	.01	.01	.4
Gooseberries, raw	½ cup	45	330	0	0	0
Gooseberries, canned in syrup	½ cup	103	0	0	0	0
*Grapefruit, raw	½ grapefruit	52	105	.05	.03	3
Grapefruit, canned in syrup	½ cup	80	10	.04	.03	3
Grapes, raw	½ cup	76	115	.06	.03	3
*Lemon, raw, peeled, med.	1 whole	19	15	.03	.01	Tr
*Lime, medium, peeled	1 whole	16	Tr	Tr	Tr	Tr
Loganberries, raw	½ cup	71	230	.04	.05	.5
Loganberries, w/syrup	½ cup	102	150	.01	.02	.2
*Melon, honeydew, medium	⅛ melon	75	85	.09	.06	1.3

	Minerals					Fatty Acids		Salt	
(Mg) Phosphorus	(Mg) Iron	(Mg) Calcium	Carbo-hydrate %	Pro-tein %	Fat %	% Satu-rated	% Unsatu-rated	(Mg) Sodium	(Mg) Potassium
1	.3	7	13.3	.2	.3	—	—	2	126
0	.5	5	19.7	.2	.2	—	—	3	62
0	.5	5	10.7	.2	.2	—	—	2	88
3	.5	17	12.2	1.0	.2	—	—	1	353
8	.4	12	21.4	.6	.1	—	—	2	74
2	.6	7	21.7	1.1	.2	—	—	3	321
22	.8	20	20.0	.7	.2	—	—	.8	0
19	.7	19	22.6	.8	.3	—	—	—	—
15	1.1	17	13.8	.7	.5	—	—	1	83
7	.6	13	25.0	.4	.4	—	—	—	—
2	5	7	25.6	.6	.3	—	—	—	—
43	1.0	41	7.2	.7	.1	—	—	35	867
2	.8	28	6.0	1.2	Tr	—	—	25	534
2	.5	25	17.0	1.3	.3	—	—	1	295
4	.4	13	25.0	.6	.2	—	—	3	62
7	.6	14	27.6	1.0	.4	—	—	1	317
7	.2	3	17.2	.4	.3	—	—	—	—
1	.6	16	9.4	.4	.7	—	—	3	88
4	.2	4	52.0	.2	.3	—	—	1	34
53	2.3	73	8.7	1.4	2	—	—	2	291
86	2.0	34	70.6	2.2	.5	—	—	1	448
13	.3	20	19.1	1.2	.3	—	—	2	329
8	2.8	140	127	4.6	2.6	—	—	39	85
5	.5	42	30.0	.7	.2	—	—	1	119
3	.4	11	18.4	.3	.3	—	—	10	181
7	.6	21	7.8	.8	.2	—	—	1	176
0	.3	12	21.8	.5	.1	—	—	4	111
1	.3	21	10.4	.5	.1	—	—	1	172
6	.4	15	18.3	.5	.2	—	—	2	—
3	.5	14	16.8	.6	.3	—	—	4.5	204
1	.4	19	7.8	1.1	.3	—	—	—	—
.9	.3	15	9.0	1.0	.3	—	—	1	14
9	1.4	40	11.9	1.0	.6	—	—	.3	291
3	.9	25	20.3	.6	.4	—	—	—	—
4	.8	30	7.1	.8	.3	—	—	—	—

Food Product	Portions	Calories	Vitamins A (I.U.)	B Group (Mg) Thiamin	Ribo-Flavin	Niacin	C Ase
*Melon, honeydew & cantaloup frozen in syrup	½ cup	71	1,760	.03	.02	6	
*Nectarines, raw	1 medium	54	1,415	0	0	0	
*Oranges	3 inch	71	285	.14	.06	.6	
*Papayas, raw	⅛ slice of papaya	45	2,000	.05	.05	.3	
*Peaches, raw	1 medium	43	1,520	.02	.06	1.1	
Peaches, w/syrup	2 halves	84	520	.01	.02	.7	
Peaches frozen in syrup	½ cup	101	740	.01	.04	.8	
Pears	1 medium	87	30	.03	.05	1	
Pears w/syrup	2 halves	78	Tr	.01	.02	.2	
Pineapple, raw medium	⅛ slice	74	80	.13	.04	.03	
Pineapple, w/syrup	½ cup	85	60	.09	.02	.2	
Plums, Damson raw	1-3 inches	66	300	.08	0.3	.5	
*Plums, prune type, raw	1-2 inches	43	170	.02	.02	.3	
Plums w/syrup	3 plums	91	1,440	.03	.03	.4	
Prunes dried, uncooked	4 prunes	196	915	.05	1.0	.9	
Prunes, softened cooked no sugar	4 prunes	145	885	.03	.08	.8	
*Pumpkin, canned	½ cup	38	7,310	.03	.06	.7	
Raisins natural, uncooked	¼ cup	164	10	.06	.05	.3	
Raspberries, black raw	½ cup	63	Tr	.02	.08	.8	
*Raspberries, red raw	½ cup	49	110	.02	.08	.8	
Raspberries, red frozen	½ cup	112	80	.02	.07	.7	2
*Strawberries, raw	½ cup	32	50	.03	.06	.6	5
Strawberries, whole, frozen	½ cup	105	35	.02	.07	.6	6
*Tangerines	½ cup	52	410	.06	.02	.1	35
Watermelon	1 inch slice from half melon 8 oz.	59	1,350	.07	.07	.5	16

Fruit Juices

Apple	¾ cup	81	0	Tr	.01	.13	
Apricot, canned 40% fruit	½ cup	65	1,085	.01	.01	.2	3
Blackberry, canned	½ cup	42	0	.02	.03	.3	11
Grape, canned	½ cup	75	0	.05	.02	.2	T

						Fatty Acids		Salt	
Minerals			Carbo-hydrate %	Pro-tein %	Fat %	% Satu-rated	% Unsatu-rated		
(g) Phosphorus	(Mg) Iron	(Mg) Calcium						(Mg) Sodium	(Mg) Potassium
4	.3	.11	15.4	.6	.1	—	—	—	—
0	.4	3	16.7	.6	Tr	—	—	5	251
1	.5	57	12.2	1.3	.1	—	—	1.4	275
8	.3	23	9.1	.6	.1	—	—	3.4	265
21	.6	10	9.1	.6	.1	—	—	5	240
3	4.0	4	19.1	.5	.1	—	—	6	35
5	6	5	22.2	.4	.1	—	—	3	136
16	.4	11	13.9	.7	.4	—	—	4	180
12	.2	9	18.1	.2	.1	—	—	2	0
1	7.1	24	13.3	.4	.2	—	—	3	309
6	.3	12	19.1	.3	.1	—	—	1	110
17	.5	18	17.4	5	Tr	—	—	2	299
10	.3	7	19.3	8	.2	—	—	1	170
16	1.2	10	20.4	4	.1	—	—	1	161
56	2.5	51	89.1	3.3	.5	—	—	9	799
45	2.2	29	65.8	2.1	.6	—	—	7	590
30	.5	29	6.6	1.0	.3	—	—	—	—
57	2.0	35	76.6	2.5	.2	—	—	18	455
19	.8	26	10.6	1.5	1.4	—	—	2.8	254
19	.8	19	10.6	1.2	.5	—	—	2.8	254
19	.7	15	22.4	.7	.2	—	—	—	—
18	.9	18	7.1	.7	.5	—	—	1.3	138
18	.7	15	22.9	.4	.2	—	—	2	204
20	.5	46	11.1	.8	.2	—	—	2.5	175
23	1.1	16	6.1	.5	.2	—	—	2	274
0	2.6	11	10.8	.1	.1	—	—	Tr	81
14.0	2	10	14.4	.3	.1	—	—	4	0
14.0	1.0	14	7.8	.3	.6	—	—	—	—
14	.3	13	16.6	.2	Tr	—	—	1	136

| | | | **Vitamins** | | | | |
Food Product	**Portions**	**Calories**	**A** (I.U.)	**B Group (Mg)** Thiamin	Ribo-Flavin	Niacin	**C** As
*Grapefruit, fresh	½ cup	45	0	.05	.02	.2	
Grapefruit, canned, sweetened	1 cup	98	0	.06	.01	.24	
Grapefruit, canned, unsweetened	1 cup	120	0	.06	.02	.13	
*Grapefruit/orange canned sweetened	½ cup	57	115	.06	.02	.2	
Grapefruit/orange canned unsweetened	½ cup	49	115	.06	.02	.2	
*Lemon, fresh	¼ cup	14	10	.02	.01	.01	
Lemon, frozen concentrate	¼ cup	64	50	.08	.04	.2	1
*Orange, fresh	½ cup	55	230	.10	.03	.5	
*Orange, frozen concentrate	diluted w/3 parts water, ½ cup	51	230	.10	.01	.3	
Pineapple, canned	½ cup	61	100	.06	.02	.2	
Prune, canned or bottled	½ cup	88	0	.01	.01	.5	
*Tangerine, fresh	½ cup	49	480	.07	.02	.1	

Vegetables

*Artichokes, cooked	½ cup	30	170	.08	.05	.8	
*Asparagus, fresh cooked	½ cup	23	1,030	.18	.21	1.6	3
*Asparagus, frozen/cooked	½ cup	25	970	.16	.15	1.1	2
Beans, white, navy, dry, cooked	½ cup	135	0	.16	.08	.8	
Beans, limas fresh cooked	½ cup	126	320	.21	.11	1.5	1
Beans, limas, frozen cooked	½ cup	136	250	.10	.06	1.4	1
Beans, red kidney, cooked or canned	½ cup	108	0	.06	.06	1.0	
*Beans, green snap fresh cooked	½ cup	29	660	.07	.08	.3	1
*Beans, green snap-frozen	½ cup	29	660	.08	.10	.5	
*Beans, yellow wax fresh, cooked	½ cup	25	260	.08	.10	.6	1
*Beans, yellow wax, frozen	½ cup	31	115	.08	.09	.5	
*Beet greens, fresh cooked	½ cup	20	5,825	.08	.17	.3	1
Beets, red, cooked or canned	½ cup	38	20	.01	.03	.01	

Minerals						Fatty Acids		Salt	
(Mg) Phosphorus	(Mg) Iron	(Mg) Calcium	Carbohydrate %	Protein %	Fat %	% Saturated	% Unsaturated	(Mg) Sodium	(Mg) Potassium
17	.2	10	9.2	.5	.1	—	—	1	184
34	7	22	9.7	.4	Tr	—	—	1	184
32	9	18	12.8	.4	Tr	—	—	1	184
17	.2	.11	12.1	.5	.1	—	—	Tr	108
17	.3	.11	10.0	.6	.2	—	—	.3	0
.6	.1	.4	16.0	.10	.4	—	—	.2	48
26	.6	18	72.8	4.6	.18	—	—	28	372
21	.2	13	11.2	.10	.1	—	—	1	227
18	.1	10	10.7	.7	.1	—	—	—	—
10	.6	18	13.0	.3	.1	—	—	1.1	160
23	4.7	16	19.0	.4	.1	—	—	.2	295
16	.2	21	10.0	.5	.2	—	—	—	—

Calcium	Phos.	Iron	Carbohydrate %	Protein %	Fat %	% Saturated	% Unsaturated	(Mg) Sodium	(Mg) Potassium
58	78	1.3	7.1	2.8	.2	—	—	49	490
24	57	.7	.9	2.2	.2	—	—	3	212
25	73	1.4	2.7	3.2	.2	—	—	2.2	0
57	169	3.0	19.7	7.8	.6	—	—	11.4	1356
54	138	2.9	18.0	7.6	.5	—	—	1	771
40	142	3.0	20.4	7.4	.2	—	—	171	0
48	149	2.3	16.4	5.6	.4	—	—	—	—
57	42	.7	3.4	1.6	.2	—	—	3	284
46	37	.8	4.7	1.6	.1	—	—	1.5	180
57	42	.7	3.6	1.4	.2	—	—	—	—
40	35	.8	5.1	1.7	.1	—	—	—	—
113	29	2.1	2.2	1.7	.2	—	—	—	—
17	34	.7	7.8	.9	.1	—	—	41	136

			Vitamins				
				B Group (Mg)			**C** (M
Food Product	**Portions**	**Calories**	**A** (I.U.)	**Thiamin**	**Ribo-Flavin**	**Niacin**	Ascor Aci
*Broccoli, cooked fresh	½ cup	30	2,855	.10	.23	.9	10:
*Broccoli, frozen	½ cup	29	2,970	.07	.14	.6	6!
*Brussel Sprouts, fresh cooked	½ cup	41	595	.09	.16	.9	99
frozen	½ cup	38	650	.09	.11	.7	92
*Cabbage, raw	½ cup	29	150	.06	.06	.3	54
Cabbage, cooked	½ cup	21	140	.02	.02	.1	27
*Cabbage, red, raw	½ cup	35	45	.10	.07	.5	70
*Cabbage, celery raw	½ cup	16	170	.06	.05	.7	29
*Carrots, raw	½ cup	48	12,560	.06	.06	.6	1
*Carrots, cooked	½ cup	35	12,000	.06	.06	.6	7
*Carrots and peas, frozen	½ cup	60	10,625	.21	.08	1.5	9
*Cauliflower, fresh cooked	½ cup	25	70	.10	.09	.7	63
*Cauliflower, raw	½ cup	31	70	.13	.11	.8	88
Celeriac Root, raw	½ cup	46	—	.06	.06	.8	10
*Celery, raw	½ cup	20	270	.02	.02	.2	10
*Celery, steamed	½ cup	16	260	.02	.03	.3	7
*Chard, raw	½ cup	29	7,425	.07	.19	.6	36
*Chard, cooked	½ cup	21	6,165	.05	.13	.5	18
*Chives, raw	1 Tbsp	4	1,660	.02	.04	.1	16
*Collard greens, cooked	½ cup	36	8,900	.10	.10	.3	72.
*Collard greens, frozen	½ cup	34	7,770	.07	.16	.7	38
Corn, yellow bantam, fresh cooked	1 ear 7 inches	123	540	.16	.14	1.8	12.
Corn kernels, frozen	½ cup	90	400	.10	.07	1.7	6.
Corn, yellow, kernel canned	½ cup	75	130	.04	.06	1.1	6.
Corn, yellow, cream style	½ cup	92	130	.04	.06	1.1	6.
Corn, white kernel canned	½ cup	70	40	.03	.05	1.1	5.
Corn, white, cream style, canned	½ cup	91	20	.03	.05	1.3	6
Cucumber, raw	7½″ long	38	Tr	.08	.11	.5	
Eggplant, boiled	½ cup	22	10	.06	.05	.6	3.
*Endive, raw	½ cup	23	3,770	.08	.16	.6	11.
*Escarole, raw	½ cup	23	3,770	.08	.16	.6	11
Garlic	1 clove	3	Tr	Tr	Tr	Tr	Tr
*Kohlrabi, raw	½ cup	44	9,480	.11	.20	1.8	106.
*Kale, fresh, cooked	½ cup	33	25	.07	.04	.3	75.
Lentils, cooked	½ cup	121	25	.08	.07	.7	0
*Lettuce (Leaf)	¼ pound	20	2,160	.06	.08	.4	20.

	Minerals						Fatty Acids		Salt	
(Mg) Calcium	(Mg) Phos.	(Mg) Iron	Carbo-hydrate %	Pro-tein %	Fat %	% Satu-rated	% Unsatu-rated	(Mg) Sodium	(Mg) Potassium
101	71	.9	3.0	3.1	.3	—	—	11	325
61	64	.8	3.5	2.9	.3	—	—	15	283
37	82	1.3	4.8	4.2	.4	—	—	10	316
24	70	.9	5.3	3.2	.2	—	—	31	—
56	33	.5	4.6	1.3	.2	—	—	22	201
48	19	.3	3.2	1.0	.2	—	—	—	—
48	40	.9	5.9	2.0	.2	—	—	—	—
49	46	.7	2.4	1.2	.1	—	—	36	342
42	42	.8	8.7	1.1	.2	—	—	58	379
38	35	.7	6.1	.9	.2	—	—	48	159
29	65	1.3	8.6	3.2	.3	—	—	80	150
24	48	.8	3.1	2.3	.2	—	—	18	—
29	64	1.3	4.2	2.7	.2	—	—	—	—
50	12	.6	14.2	3.6	.6	—	—	—	—
44	32	.4	3.3	.9	.1	—	—	124	340
35	25	.2	2.5	.8	.1	—	—	—	—
101	45	3.6	3.8	2.4	.3	—	—	125	625
83	27	2.0	2.6	1.8	.2	—	—	—	—
20	13	.5	4.7	1.8	.3	—	—	—	—
208	57	.9	3.9	3.5	.7	—	—	49	456
201	58	1.1	4.6	2.9	.4	—	—	—	—
4	120	.8	20.3	3.3	1.0	—	—	11	215
3	83	.9	18.3	3.0	.5	—	—	10	205
4	57	.4	15.5	1.9	.6	—	—	238	227
4	66	.7	19.2	2.1	.6	—	—	—	—
5	52	.5	14.1	1.9	.6	—	—	—	—
3	63	.7	18.8	2.2	.6	—	—	—	—
46	49	.8	2.9	.6	.1	—	—	16	442
13	24	.7	3.2	1.0	.2	—	—	4	215
93	62	1.9	3.2	1.7	.1	—	—	20	455
93	62	1.9	3.2	1.7	.1	—	—	20	455
1	5	Tr	29.3	6.2	.2	—	—	—	—
214	65	1.8	6.1	4.5	.7	—	—	94	430
47	58	.6	5.6	2.0	.1	—	—	11	382
29	136	2.4	18.1	7.8	Tr	—	—	3	1860
78	28	.16	2.8	1.3	.3	—	—	3.4	236

Food Product	Portions	Calories	A (I.U.)	Thiamin	Ribo-Flavin	Niacin	C (Ascorbic Ac...)
*Lettuce, head	¼ head	14	360	.06	.06	.4	
Mixed vegetables, frozen (carrots, corn, peas, beans, limas)	½ cup	73	5,660	.14	.08	1.3	
*Mushrooms, canned	½ cup	19	Tr	.02	.29	2.2	
*Mushrooms, raw	½ cup	32	Tr	.11	.53	4.8	
*Mustard greens, fresh cooked	½ cup	26	6,625	.09	.16	.7	
Mustard greens, frozen	½ cup	23	6,855	.03	.11	1.0	
*Okra, boiled fresh	½ cup	33	560	.15	.21	1.0	
*Okra, frozen	½ cup	43	550	.16	.19	1.1	
Onions, raw	½ cup	43	45	.03	.05	.2	
Onions, dehydrated flaked	¼ cup	220	120	1.4	1.0	.80	
Parsely, raw	1 tbsp	13	Tr	Tr	Tr	Tr	
Parsnips, fresh, cooked	½ cup	75	35	.08	.09	.10	
Peas, blackeye or cowpeas	½ cup	123	400	.34	.13	1.6	
Peas (chick, garbanzos), raw, dried	½ cup	411	60	.35	.17	2.3	
*Peas, green, cooked fresh	½ cup	81	615	.32	.13	2.6	2
*Peas, green, frozen	½ cup	78	685	.31	.10	1.9	1
Peas, split, dry raw	½ cup	395	135	.85	.33	3.4	
*Peas, green, canned	½ cup	60	510	.14	.06	1.2	1
*Peppers (sweet, green) raw	½ cup	26	480	1.0	1.0	.6	14
*Peppers (sweet, red) raw	½ cup	36	506.0	1.0	1.0	.6	23
*Peppers (sweet) canned	½ cup	20	2,795	.02	.06	.6	9
*Pimientoes, canned	1 medium	8	810	.01	.03	.2	4
Potatoes, baked in skin	1 small	106	Tr	.11	.05	.19	2
Potatoes, boiled in skin	1 small	87	Tr	.10	.05	1.7	1
Potatoes, boiled w/out skin	1 small	74	Tr	.10	.03	1.4	1
Potatoes, french fried	½ cup	313	Tr	.15	1.09	3.5	2
Potatoes, mashed	½ cup	106	160	.07	.05	.8	
Potatoes, dehydrated flakes	½ cup	415	Tr	.26	.07	6.2	3
Radishes, raw	½ cup	20	10	.04	.04	.4	1
Rhubarb, cooked sweetened	1 cup	385	70	Tr	0	.2	

| Minerals | | | Carbo-hydrate % | Pro-tein % | Fat % | Fatty Acids | | Salt | |
(Mg) Calcium	(Mg) Phos.	(Mg) Iron				% Satu-rated	% Unsatu-rated	(Mg) Sodium	(Mg) Potassium
22	24	.6	2.4	.9	.1	—	—	40	—
29	72	1.5	12.2	3.2	.3	—	—	67	236
7	78	.6	1.8	1.9	.1	—	—	85	404
7	132	.9	3.6	2.7	.3	—	—	8	560
159	37	2.0	3.1	2.2	.4	—	—	39	447
119	49	1.7	2.1	2.2	.4	—	—	85	454
105	47	.6	5.0	2.0	.3	—	—	1	249
107	49	.6	7.8	2.2	.1	—	—	—	—
31	41	.6	8.1	1.5	.1	—	—	8	84
94	142	1.6	77.7	8.7	1.3	—	—	—	—
56	18	1.8	7.0	3.6	.6	—	—	13	206
51	71	.7	12.9	1.5	.5	—	—	9	529
27	167	2.4	16.3	8.1	.8	—	—	40	1,110
172	377	7.9	56.0	20.5	4.8	—	—	45	1,210
26	113	2.1	10.1	5.4	.4	—	—	5	357
22	98	2.2	9.9	5.1	.3	—	—	113	181
38	306	5.8	61.5	24.2	1.0	—	—	48	998
22	67	1.7	8.9	3.4	.4	—	—	2	—
10	26	.8	3.4	1.2	.2	—	—	1.2	200
14	34	.6	5.4	1.4	.3	—	—	1.2	200
3	13.7	1.4	6.0	.8	.5	—	—	—	—
3	12	1.0	4.7	.7	.2	—	—	—	—
10	74	.8	20.5	2.6	.1	—	—	5	496
8	61	.7	16.6	2.1	1.1	—	—	4	385
7	48	.6	14.0	1.9	.1	—	—	9	465
17	127	1.5	35.0	4.3	13.2	—	—	4	496
29	48	1.4	15.3	1.8	2.8	—	—	90	260
40	198	1.9	82.4	7.2	.6	—	—	100	1,814
34	36	1.2	2.9	1.0	.1	—	—	10	294
39	112	1.1	98	.1	Tr	—	—	15	510

Food Product	Portions	Calories	Vitamins A (I.U.)	B Group (Mg) Thiamin	Ribo-Flavin	Niacin	C (M Ascor Aci)
Rutabagas, cooked	½ cup	40	625	.07	.07	.9	30.0
Sauerkraut, canned	½ cup	21	50	.04	.07	.1	18.0
*Spinach, raw	½ cup	30	9,255	.11	.23	.7	58.0
*Spinach, frozen	½ cup	26	9,025	.08	.17	.5	22.0
Soy beans, cooked	½ cup	130	30	.2	.05	.6	—
*Squash, acorn baked	½ cup	63	1,600	.06	.15	.8	15.0
*Squash, acorn, boiled	½ cup	39	1,255	.05	.11	.5	9.0
*Squash, butternut baked	½ cup	78	7,310	.06	.15	.8	9.0
Squash, butternut boiled	½ cup	47	6,170	.05	.11	.5	6.0
Squash, winter or hubbard baked	½ cup	72	4,800	.06	.15	.8	15.0
*Squash, winter or hubbard boiled	½ cup	43	4,000	.05	.11	.5	9.0
Squash, yellow, frozen	½ cup	24	160	.07	.05	.5	9.0
Succotash, frozen	½ cup	106	340	.10	.06	1.5	7.0
Sweet Potatoes baked in skin	1 medium	190	9,200	.15	.11	1.0	28.0
Sweet Potatoes, boiled	1 medium	160	9,105	.10	.07	.08	22.2
Sweet Potatoes, candied	1 medium	235	9,000	.8	.06	1.1	29.0
*Tomatoes, raw	1 medium 2″ x 2″	25	1,800	.07	.05	.9	26.0
*Tomatoes, boiled	½ cup	30	1,740	.08	.06	.9	27.0
*Tomatoes, canned	½ cup	24	1,600	.06	.04	.8	20.0
Turnips, cooked	½ cup	26	Tr	.04	.06	.3	25.0
*Turnip greens, cooked	½ cup	22	6,510	.11	.26	.6	54.0
*Watercress, raw	¼ bunch	5	1,400	.02	.05	.2	23.0
*Zucchini, raw	½ cup	19	365	.06	.10	1.1	22.0
Zucchini, cooked	½ cup	14	340	.06	.09	.9	10.0

Vegetable Juices

Food Product	Portions	Calories	Vitamins A (I.U.)	B Group (Mg) Thiamin	Ribo-Flavin	Niacin	C (M Ascor Aci)
*Sauerkraut juice, canned	½ cup	11	—	.03	.05	.2	22.0
*Tomato juice, canned	½ cup	22	910	.06	.03	.9	18.0
*Vegetable cocktail	½ cup	19	1,285	.06	.03	.9	20.0

Meat
Beef

Food Product	Portions	Calories	Vitamins A (I.U.)	B Group (Mg) Thiamin	Ribo-Flavin	Niacin	C (M Ascor Aci)
Bottom Round, (choice grade), raw	¼ pound	347	107	.09	.18	4.9	—
Steak, Sirloin	¼ pound	440	66	Tr	Tr	5	0

	Minerals					Fatty Acids		Salt	
(Mg) Calcium	(Mg) Phos.	(Mg) Iron	Carbo-hydrate %	Pro-tein %	Fat %	% Satu-rated	% Unsatu-rated	(Mg) Sodium	(Mg) Potassium
67	35	.3	7.1	.9	.1	—	—	6	287
39	20	.6	3.8	1.1	.3	—	—	687	153
106	58	3.5	3.7	3.2	.3	—	—	95	569
129	50	2.4	2.9	3.0	.3	—	—	48	235
75	180	2.9	10 grs	11 grs.	5.5 grs.	—	—	2	540
45	33	1.3	12.2	1.9	.1	—	—	—	—
46	82	1.1	7.0	1.2	.1	—	—	—	—
46	80	1.1	15.7	1.8	.1	—	—	—	—
33	56	.8	9.0	1.1	.1	—	—	—	—
32	55	.9	13.6	1.8	.4	—	—	—	—
23	37	.6	7.8	1.1	3	—	—	1	255
16	37	.8	4.1	1.4	.1	—	—	—	—
15	97	1.1	19.6	4.2	.4	—	—	51	310
45	66	1.0	31.6	2.1	5	—	—	12	300
47	60	1.0	25.6	1.7	.4	—	—	16	300
50	70	1.6	80 grs	2 grs.	6 grs.	—	—	18	360
15	31	.6	4.2	1.1	.2	—	—	3.2	327
17	37	.7	4.9	1.3	.2	—	—	3.1	300
7	22	.6	3.9	1.0	.2	—	—	20	147
40	27	.4	4.0	.8	.2	—	—	—	—
199	39	1.1	2.6	2.2	.2	—	—	—	—
43	15	.5	2.3	2.2	.3	—	—	—	—
32	33	.5	3.0	1.2	.1	—	—	—	—
29	29	.5	1.9	1.0	.1	—	—	—	—
42	16	1.3	2.3	.7	Tr	—	—	—	—
8	20	1.0	4.1	.9	.1	—	—	6	261
14	25	.6	3.1	.9	.1	—	—	21	—
11	133	3.0	0	17.4	25.3	12 grs	Tr	145	450
10	200	3.3	0	27 grs.	36 grs.	31 "	1 gr.	80	429

Food Product	Portions	Calories	A (I.U.)	B Group (Mg) Thiamin	B Group (Mg) Ribo-Flavin	B Group (Mg) Niacin	C (Mg) Ascorbic Acid
Steak, Ground lean	¼ pound	177	30	Tr	Tr	8.1	0
Hamburger (commercial)	¼ pound	367	40	Tr	Tr	7.9	0
Rib Roast Beef, Oven cooked	¼ pound	520	80	Tr	Tr	4	0
Chuck, boneless (choice grade), raw	¼ pound	402	67	.08	.16	.45	0
*Flank steak	¼ pound	164	12.5	.10	.21	5.6	0
Porterhouse Steak w/out fat, broiled	¼ pound	262	23	.09	.26	7.0	0
T-Bone Steak (choice, w/out fat)	¼ pound	255	23	.09	.26	7.1	0
*Beef Liver	¼ pound	160	**	.26	3.83	15.8	71.0
*Calves Liver	¼ pound	160	**	.23	3.1	13.0	41.0
Corned Beef, Cooked	¼ pound	424	0	.2	.27	1.7	0
Tongue, smoked cooked	¼ pound	305	0	.06	.33	4.0	0
*Beef kidney	¼ pound	147	785	.27	2.91	7.3	34.0
*Veal kidney (Baby Beef)	¼ pound	129	—	—	—	—	13.0
*Lamb kidney	¼ pound	120	790	.53	2.75	8.5	17.0
Calves Sweetbreads	¼ pound	192	—	.07	.18	3.3	—
Calves brains	½ pound	150	—	.3	2.5	4.9	—

Lamb

Food Product	Portions	Calories	A (I.U.)	Thiamin	Ribo-Flavin	Niacin	Ascorbic Acid
Leg, roasted	¼ pound	365	—	.16	.26	6.5	—
Loin chop, broiled	¼ pound	410	—	.16	.23	5.3	—
Rib chop, broiled	¼ pound	465	—	.13	.44	5.3	—
Shoulder chop, broiled	¼ pound	386	—	.15	.26	5.7	—

Pork

Food Product	Portions	Calories	A (I.U.)	Thiamin	Ribo-Flavin	Niacin	Ascorbic Acid
Bacon, broiled or fried	2 slices	97	0	Tr	Tr	.8	0
Ham, canned	¼ pound	220	0	.61	.22	4.3	—
Ham, Med. Fat— Light Cure	¼ pound	322	0	.82	.22	4.7	—
Loin Roast or Chops	¼ pound	413	0	1.04	.30	6.4	0
Salt Pork	¼ pound	894	0	.20	.04	1	—
Spareribs	¼ pound	412	0	.80	.19	4.3	—

** Liver varies widely from 100 I.U. vitamin A to more than 100.000 I.U. per ¼ pound

| Minerals | | | | | | Fatty Acids | | Salt | |
Calcium (Mg)	Phos. (Mg)	Iron (Mg)	Carbohydrate %	Protein %	Fat %	% Saturated	% Unsaturated	Sodium (Mg)	Potassium (Mg)
12.5	202	4	0	3.2 "	15 "	12 "	Tr "	143	452
12	197	3.2	0	28 "	24 "	20 "	Tr "	133	426
9	138	3	0	21.5 "	48 "	47 "	Tr "	80	480
10	170	3.0	0	18.7	19.6	10 "	Tr "	76	390
16	230	3.1	0	21.7	5.4	12 "	Tr "	140	450
13	275	4.2	0	30.2	10.5	20 "	1 "	80	425
13	277	4.2	0	15.2	10.3	25 "	1 "	60	320
9	402	7.4	4.1	19.2	4.7	Tr "	Tr "	184	331
.09	387	10	3.8	19.2	4.7	— "	— "	125	431
10	106	3.3	0	22.9	30.4	9 "	Tr "	1200	60
—	—	—	.3	19.3	20.3	7 grs.	Tr	81	214
13	240	8.5	.9	16.6	6.7	—	—	2075	2070
—	—	9.0	.1	16.6	4.6	—	—	—	—
15	249	8.6	.9	16.8	3.3	—	—	283	288
—	—	—	0	32.6	3.2	—	—	121	372
12	337	2.9	0	12.5 grs.	8.5 grs.	—	—	130	240
12.5	241	2.05	0	23.9	12.0	—	—	—	—
10.05	185	1.5	0	22.0	14.9	—	—	103	387
10.05	178	1.3	0	20.1	35.6	—	—	103	387
12	195	1.3	0	21.7	27.2	—	—	103	387
2	42	5	3.2	30.4	52.0	7 "	1 "	600	65
12	177	3.1	.9	18.3	12.3	5 "	1 "	1399	253
11	185	3.0	0	17.5	23.5	9 "	2 "	1270	391
13	291	3.6	0	24.5	28.5	10 grs.	2 grs.	40	360
Tr	Tr	.6	0	3.9	85.0	—	—	—	—
9	183	2.5	0	14.5	33.2	14 "	3 "	—	—

Vitamins

Food Product	Portions	Calories	A (I.U.)	B Group (Mg) Thiamin	Ribo-Flavin	Niacin	C (Mg) Ascorbic Acid
Veal							
Veal cutlet, broiled	¼ pound	265	0	Tr	.3	7	0
Veal roast, baked	¼ pound	400	0	.15	.4	7.3	0
Rabbit	¼ pound	184	—	.09	.07	14.6	—
Chicken							
*Broiled chicken	½ pound	210	340	Tr	.3	17	0
*Chicken livers (fried)	3 medium	140	**32,200	.2	2.4	11.8	20
Chicken, roasted	½ pound	662	2,190	.16	.50	16.8	0
Turkey							
Roasted	½ pound	601	—	1.1	.44	17.1	—
Dairy Products							
Cow's milk whole	1 qt.	660	1,560	.32	1.7	.8	
*Cow's milk, skimmed	1 qt.	360	***	.4	1.7	.8	
*Yogurt, part skim milk	1 cup	120	170	.1	.4	.2	
Custard, baked	1 cup	131	870	.1	.5	.2	
Ice cream, commercial	1 cup	300	740	Tr	.3	.1	
Ice milk commercial	1 cup	275	390	.1	.4	.2	
Evaporated skimmed	1 cup	387	Tr	.26	1.7	.92	
Buttermilk	1 cup	82	180	.1	.4	.2	
Cottage cheese, uncreamed	1 cup	195	20	.1	.6	.1	
Cheddar or American	1 inch cube	70	230	Tr	.1	Tr	
Roquefort type	1 inch cube	105	350	Tr	.2	.1	
Swiss	1 inch cube	105	320	Tr	.1	Tr	
*Eggs, boiled or poached	2 eggs (medium size)	150	1,180	Tr	.3	Tr	
Eggs, scrambled	2 eggs (medium size)	220	1,200	Tr	.4	Tr	
Butter	1 tablesp	100	460	0	Tr	0	

**Liver varies widely from 100 I.U. vitamin A to more than 100,000 I.U. per ¼ pound
***Most commercial skim milk today is fortified with 2000 I.U. vitamin A per quart.

Minerals						Fatty Acids		Salt	
(Mg) Calcium	(Mg) Phos.	(Mg) Iron	Carbo-hydrate %	Pro-tein %	Fat %	% Satu-rated	% Unsatu-rated	(Mg) Sodium	(Mg) Potassium
11	300	3.4	0	23 grs.	8.4 grs.	8 grs.	Tr	80	460
14	255	3.4	0	27.1	11.1	13	Tr	101	510
23	402	1.5	0	21.0	8	—	—	39	454
15	320	1.4	0	23.8 grs.	3.8 grs.	17 grs.	5	110	416
16	240	7.4	2.3 grs.	15.0 "	2.8 "	12 "	2	51	160
23	503	4.3	0	23.8 "	3.8 "	33 "	8	130	700
—	—	—	0	20.1 "	22.1 "	—	—	73	357
1,140	930	.4	48 grs.	32 grs.	40 grs.	36 grs.	Tr	75	210
1,192	940	.4	52 "	36 "	Tr	Tr	0	78	215
295	270	.1	13 "	8 "	4 "	3 "	Tr	19	50
278	370	1.0	28 "	13 "	14 "	11 "	1	60	100
175	150	.1	29 "	6 "	18 "	16 "	1	140	170
290	250	.1	32 grs.	9 "	10 grs.	9 grs.	Tr	58	54
388	1253	5.5	58 "	40 "	Tr	Tr	0	100	280
275	216	Tr	5.1	3.6	.1	4 grs.	Tr	19	52
202	380	.9	6 grs.	38 grs.	Tr	Tr	Tr	620	180
133	128	.1	Tr	4 "	6 grs.	5 "	Tr	180	30
122	100	.2	Tr	6 "	9 "	8 "	Tr	284	22
270	140	.2	Tr	7 "	8 "	7 "	Tr	225	25
54	205	2.3	Tr	12 "	12 "	10 "	1 gr.	122	129
60	222	2.2	Tr	13 "	16 "	14 "	1 "	338	140
3	0	Tr	Tr	Tr	11 "	10 "	Tr	120	4

Food Product	Portions	Calories	A (I.U.)	Thiamin	Ribo-Flavin	Niacin	C (Mg) Ascorbic Acid
Variety Meats							
Knockwurst	2 sausages ¼ pound	252	—	1.8	1	3	—
Liverwurst	¼ pound	264	5,720	.4	1.2	4.6	
Frankfurters	2 sausages ¼ pound	246	0	.1	.2	2.5	
Chile con carne w/beans	½ cup	167	—	.04	.09	1.8	—
Fish & Shell Fish							
Trout-Brook, raw	½ pound	230	—		.16	—	—
Lake Trout, raw	½ pound	384	—	.20	.27	6.2	—
Halibut, broiled	½ pound	390	1,055	.11	.16	18.9	—
White Fish Lake, raw	½ pound	353	5,200	.32	.27	6.8	
White Fish Lake, smoked	¼ pound	177	—	—	—	—	—
*Snapper red, raw	¼ pound	110	—	.15	.2	—	—
Salmon, canned	½ cup	177	200	.04	.19	8.7	—
Salmon, smoked	¼ pound	200	—	—	—	—	
Tuna, canned in oil	½ cup	328	100	.04	.11	11.1	
*Scallops, small bay, raw	½ cup	92	—	—	.07	1.5	
*Clams, fresh, raw	6 medium	102	—	.01	.12	1.0	
*Oysters, raw	6 or 8 med. or ½ cup	85	320	.2	.2	3.3	0
*Lobster, steamed	½ average size	92	0	.1	Tr	1.9	0
Oils-Fats-Dressings							
Hydrogenated cooking fat	1½ cup	665	0	0	0	0	0
Margarine	½ cup ¼ pound	806	3,700	0	Tr	0	0
Corn Oil	1 tablesp	101	0	0	0	0	0
Soy Oil	1 tablesp	101	0	0	0	0	0
Peanut Oil	1 tablesp	101	0	0	0	0	0
Cottonseed Oil	1 tablesp	101	0	0	0	0	0
Olive Oil	1 tablesp	101	0	0	0	0	0
Mayonnaise	1 tablesp	110	40	Tr	Tr	Tr	0
Sugars & Syrups							
White granulated sugar	½ cup	374	0	0	0	0	0

Minerals						Fatty Acids		Salt	
(Mg) Calcium	(Mg) Phos.	(Mg) Iron	Carbo-hydrate %	Pro-tein %	Fat %	% Unsatu-rated	% Satu-rated	(Mg) Sodium	(Mg) Potassium
10	164	2.2	2.2	14.8	23.2	1	18	1100	217
8	240	—	2 grs.	16 grs.	22 grs.	—	—	900	150
6	50	1.2	4 "	14 "	20 "	1	18	1000	215
44	175	1.6	8.4	6.4	9.4	Tr	7	530	250
—	606	—	0	19.2%	2.1%	Tr	7	—	—
—	545	1.8	0	18.3 "	10.0 "	—	9	—	—
36	568	1.8	0	25.2 "	7.0 "	—	—	127	771
—	616	.9	0	18.9 "	8.2 "	—	—	118	688
25	312	—	0	20.9 "	7.3 "	—	—	—	—
19	298	1.0	0	19.8 "	.9 "	—	—	—	—
255	350	1.1	0	20.4 "	6.9 "	Tr	5	696	446
16	280	—	0	22.2 "	18.3 "	—	—	—	—
7	332	.5	0	24.2 "	20.5 "	9	8	1207	454
30	236	2.0	3.3	15.3 "	.2 "	—	—	289	449
88	194	9.6	5.9	11.1 "	.9 "	—	—	170	230
113	150	6.6	3 grs.	8 grs.	2 grs.	0	0	80	120
65	65	.6	Tr	18 "	1 "	0	0	180	192
0	0	0	0	0	100 grs.	7 grs.	88 grs.	4	0
22	16	0	Tr	Tr	91 "	8 "	76 "	1050	58
0	0	0	0	0	14 grs.	7 grs.	5 grs.	0	0
0	0	0	0	0	—	7 "	5 "	0	0
0	0	0	0	0	—	7 "	5 "	0	0
0	—	0	0	0	14 grs.	1 "	13 "	0	0
2	8	.1	Tr	Tr	12 "	6 "	5 "	85	3
0	0	.1	99.5	0	0	—	—	—	—

Food Product	Portions	Calories	Vitamins A (I.U.)	B Group (Mg) Thiamin	B Group (Mg) Ribo-Flavin	B Group (Mg) Niacin	C (Mg) Ascorb Acid
Brown sugar	½ cup	428	0	Tr	Tr	Tr	0
Maple syrup	½ cup	288	—	—	.12	Tr	0
Honey strained	½ cup	480	0	Tr	Tr	Tr	8
Saccharin		**N O F O O D V A L U E**					

Breads & Crackers

Food Product	Portions	Calories	A (I.U.)	Thiamin	Ribo-Flavin	Niacin	Ascorb Acid
Cracked Wheat	1 slice-1 oz	75	Tr	.3	.2	.40	Tr
French or Vienna	1 slice-1 oz	82	Tr	.08	.06	.70	Tr
Raisin Bread	1 slice-1 oz	75	Tr	.01	.02	.20	Tr
Rye Bread	1 slice-1 oz	69	0	.05	.02	.4	0
White Bread	1 slice-1 oz	77	Tr	.7	.5	1.20	Tr
Whole Wheat Bread	1 slice-1 oz	68	Tr	.07	.03	.80	Tr
Graham Crackers	2 medium	55	0	Tr	Tr	.2	0
Soda Crackers	2½ inch square	45	0	Tr	Tr	.1	0

Cereal

Food Product	Portions	Calories	A (I.U.)	Thiamin	Ribo-Flavin	Niacin	Ascorb Acid
Rice, Brown	1 cup	748	0	.6	.1	9.2	0
Rice, White	1 cup	677	0	.3	Tr	7.6	0
Oatmeal	1 cup	150	0	.2	Tr	.4	0

Miscellaneous

Food Product	Portions	Calories	A (I.U.)	Thiamin	Ribo-Flavin	Niacin	Ascorb Acid
Olives, green canned, large	10	72	200	Tr	0	0	0
Olives (ripe, canned) large	10	105	60	Tr	Tr	0	0
Pickles (bread & butter)	⅛ cup	20	40	40	Tr	Tr	6.4
Pickles (dill)	5 inch-3½ oz	11	100	Tr	.02	Tr	6.0
Pickles (sour)	1 inch-1 oz	3	30	Tr	Tr	Tr	2.0
Pickles (sweet)	1 inch-1 oz	42	25	Tr	Tr	Tr	2.0
Vinegar	⅛ cup	8	—	—	—	—	0
Horseradish (prepared)	1 tablesp	5	—	—	—	—	—
Mustard Yellow	1 teasp	5	—	—	—	—	—
Tomato Catsup	2 tablesp	30	—	—	—	—	—
Tomato Chili Sauce	2 tablesp	30	—	—	—	—	—
Peanut butter	2 tablesp	200	—	.02	.02	2.7	—
Nuts, Almond (unsalted dry)	1 oz	170	0	Tr	Tr	.6	0
Brazil Nuts (unsalted)	½ cup	457	Tr	.6	.1	1.0	0

	Minerals						Fatty Acids		Salt	
(Mg) Calcium	(Mg) Phos.	(Mg) Iron	Carbo- hydrate %	Pro- tein %	Fat %	% Unsatu- rated	% Satu- rated	(Mg) Sodium	(Mg) Potassium
92	20	4.0	96.4	0	0	—	—	—	—
72	8	1.2	68.0	0	0	—	—	—	—
8	8	1.6	120 grs.	Tr	0	0	0	8	88

N O   F O O D   V A L U E

25	36	.3	51.6	8.1	2.2	0	1	52	38
12	24	.6	55.2	9.1	3.0	—	—	164	25
21	24	.6	52.7	6.6	2.8	—	—	104	67
21	42	.4	51.7	9.1	1.1	—	—	157	41
20	25	.7	50.2	8.7	3.2	—	—	144	24
28	64	.6	46.1	10.5	3.0	—	—	190	63
3	56	.3	10	1	1	—	—	90	45
2	19	.1	8	1	1	—	—	110	12

78	608	4	154 grs.	15 grs.	3 grs.	—	—	18	310
46	258	1.6	150 "	14 "	Tr "	—	—	6	300
21	140	1.7	26 "	5 "	3 "	—	—	508	142

65	13	1.2	3 grs.	1 gr.	10 grs.	—	—	1400	45
56	11	1.1	1 "	1 "	13 "	—	—	650	23
9	8	.5	17.4	.9	.2	—	—	191	—
48	—	2.6	1.5	.7	.2	—	—	1428	200
5	4	.9	1.5	.5	.2	—	—	767	—
3	5	.3	36.5	.8	.4	—	—	299	—
1	3	.2	5.9	Tr	0	—	—	—	—
9	6	Tr	8.7	1.3	.2	—	—	—	—
4	4	Tr	5.4	4.7	4.4	—	—	—	—
6	14	.2	24.9	2.0	.4	—	—	369	226
6	15	.2	24.1	2.5	.3	—	—	—	—
12	—	.3	15.1	30	50	—	—	—	—
66	144	1.3	16.9	18.6	54.2	3	1	1	220
124	464	2.3	7 grs.	10 grs.	47 grs.	12	31	1	476

Food Product	Portions	Calories	A (I.U.)	B Group (Mg) Thiamin	Ribo-Flavin	Niacin	C (M Ascor Aci
Coconut shredded (sweetened)	½ cup	274	0	Tr	Tr	Tr	
Peanuts (roasted)	½ cup	290	0	.2	.1	8.6	
Pecans raw	½ cup	343	60	.4	.1	.4	
Sesame Seeds dry	½ cup	280	15	.4	.1	2.7	
Sunflower	½ cup	280	0	1.8	.2	13.6	
Walnuts, English	½ cup	325	15	.1	.1	.4	

Beverages

Food Product	Portions	Calories	A (I.U.)	Thiamin	Ribo-Flavin	Niacin	C
Distilled Spirits— 86 proof	1 oz.	86	0	0	0	0	0
Beer	1 cup	228	0	Tr	Tr	.1	0
Dessert Wine	½ cup-4 oz	164	0	Tr	Tr	.1	0
Table Wine (dry)	½ cup	100	0	Tr	Tr	.1	0
Coffee (black)	1 cup	0	0	0	Tr	.6	0
Tea (unsweetened)	1 cup	0	0	0	Tr	Tr	0
Club Soda	12 oz- 1½ cups	0	0	0	0	0	0
Cola drinks	12 oz.	137	0	0	0	0	0
Fruit Flavored drinks	12 oz.	161	0	0	0	0	0
Root Beer	12 oz.	140	0	0	0	0	0
Ginger Ale	12 oz.	105	0	0	0	0	0
Quinine Water	8 oz-1 cup	70	0	0	0	0	0

Desserts

Food Product	Portions	Calories	A (I.U.)	Thiamin	Ribo-Flavin	Niacin	C
Custard Baked	1 cup	285	870	.1	.5	.2	T
Gelatine, Flavored	1 cup	155	0	0	0	0	0
Cake—Angel Food (Plain)	1 2-inch cube	110	0	Tr	Tr	.1	0
Sponge Cake (Plain)	1 2-inch slice	115	210	Tr	Tr	.1	0
Chocolate Cake Fudge Icing	1 2-inch cube	420	140	Tr	.1	.3	0
Gingerbread	1 2-inch slice	180	50	Tr	Tr	.6	0
Apple Pie	1 slice–1/6 of pie	330	280	Tr	Tr	.3	1
Cherry Pie	1 slice–1/6 of pie	340	520	Tr	Tr	.3	2
Custard Pie	1 slice–1/6 of pie	265	300	Tr	.2	.4	0
Lemon Meringue Pie	1 slice–1/6 of pie	300	210	Tr	.1	.2	1
Pumpkin Pie	1 slice–1/6 of pie	265	2,480	Tr	.1	.4	8

(Mg) Calcium	(Mg) Phos.	(Mg) Iron	Carbo-hydrate %	Pro-tein %	Fat %	% Saturated	% Unsaturated	(Mg) Sodium	(Mg) Potassium
						Fatty Acids		**Salt**	
8	56	1	26 "	1 "	20 "	Tr	19	0	176
37	200	1	9 "	13 "	25 "	7	16	2	337
36	144	1.2	7 "	5 "	35 "	7	25	Tr	300
580	308	5.2	10 "	9 "	24 "	10	13	30	360
60	418	3.5	10 "	12 "	26 "	15	7	15	460
50	190	1.5	8 "	7 "	32 "	20	7	1	225
0	0	0	0	Tr	0	—	—	Tr	Tr
10	60	Tr	8	Tr	0	—	—	14	50
4	Tr	Tr	9 grs.	Tr	0	0	0	2	37
10	12	.5	5 "	Tr	0	0	0	6	100
9	9	.2	1 "	Tr	0	0	0	—	—
Tr	Tr	Tr	1 "	0	Tr	0	0	Tr	—
0	—	0	0	0	0	0	0	—	—
0	—	—	—	—	0	0	0	—	—
0	0	—	38 grs. 42 grs.	0	0	0	0	—	—
0	—	—	35 "	0	0	0	0	—	—
—	0	—	25 "	0	0	0	0	—	—
0	0	0	8.0	0	0	0	0	—	—
278	370	1	28 grs.	13 grs.	14 grs.	1 gr.	11 grs.	60	100
0	0	0	36 "	4 "	Tr "	0	Tr "	122	0
2	40	.1	23 "	3 "	Tr "	—	—	113	40
11	49	.6	22 "	3 "	2 "	Tr "	2 "	70	30
118	162	.5	70 "	5 "	14 "	1 "	12 "	282	184
63	33	1.4	28 "	2 "	7 "	Tr	6 "	119	222
9	29	.5	53 "	3 "	13 "	1 "	11 "	400	106
14	33	.5	55 "	3 "	13 "	1 "	11 "	405	140
162	151	1.6	34 "	7 "	11 "	1 "	10 "	382	182
24	65	.6	45 "	4 "	12 "	1 "	10 "	337	66
70	92	1	34 "	5 "	12 "	1 "	11 "	285	219

Your Own Special Recipes

IN THE PRECEDING pages, *Staying Slim the Natural Way* has given you the basic psychological, culinary, and scientific information you need for a pleasurable and personalized program to decrease your weight and increase your joy of living.

As you translate this program into action, you will unquestionably encounter tempting new or unfamiliar dishes that with a little imagination and experiment can be made to meet your personal requirements.

If you are serious about your program, do not let these new opportunities for mealtime pleasure and caloric economy escape you. Use the following pages to note the special low-calory, high-nutrient dishes, sauces, seasonings — and in general all the tricks of slimming kitchen know-how — that will fortify *your* program.

Staying Slim the Natural Way has blazed your trail, but it is up to you to enlarge the scope and maintain the interest of your personal cuisine.